THE RUNNER'S GUIDE TO A
HEALTHY
CORE

THE RUNNER'S GUIDE TO A
HEALTHY
CORE

HOW TO STRENGTHEN THE ENGINE THAT POWERS YOUR RUNNING

DANIEL J. FREY, DPT, CMP, CSCS

FOREWORD BY CHRIS SOLINSKY

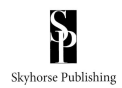

Skyhorse Publishing

Skyhorse Publishing books may be purchased in bulk at special discounts for sales promotion, corporate gifts, fund-raising, or educational purposes. Special editions can also be created to specifications. For details, contact the Special Sales Department, Skyhorse Publishing, 307 West 36th Street, 11th Floor, New York, NY 10018 or info@ skyhorsepublishing.com.

Skyhorse® and Skyhorse Publishing® are registered trademarks of Skyhorse Publishing, Inc.®, a Delaware corporation.

Visit our website at www.skyhorsepublishing.com.

10 9 8 7 6 5 4 3 2 1

Library of Congress Cataloging-in-Publication Data is available on file.

All photos by Steven Fairfield
All illustrations by Rebecca Frey

Cover design by Tom Lau
Cover photo credit: Steven Fairfield

Print ISBN: 978-1-5107-1138-9
Ebook ISBN: 978-1-5107-1139-6

Printed in China

Contents

Foreword

I have been lucky enough to experience this great sport of running from a number of vantage points. I started out as a middle school and then a high school runner before continuing on at the University of Wisconsin, where I won five NCAA titles. I was then lucky enough to run professionally for Nike for nine years, during which time I became the first American to break 27:00 for 10,000 meters and made two world championship teams. I had hoped my professional career would last longer, but it was derailed by a severe hamstring injury. I have since gotten into collegiate coaching, first at the University of Portland and now at the College of William and Mary.

As a professional runner who had his career cut short and now as a coach wanting the best for my athletes, I know and appreciate the importance of having a strong and healthy core. I often sell this notion to my athletes as working on their "beach body," but I know it is much more than that. A runner's success is closely tied to the functional strength of his or her core.

I have been asked over and over what the "secret" to success in distance running is. My answer has always been, and will always be, consistency. There are no secrets or shortcuts in running; just pure day-in, day-out running. To improve as a runner you have to run, recover, repeat. There are many different levels of this, and you can have success at any degree of this model, but it will always boil down to run, recover, repeat.

When injuries occur, they disrupt this cycle, which then prevents improvement. That's why every runner out there at any level is in pursuit of what will keep them healthy—they try new shoes, fancy gadgets, specialists, and countless books. What ended my professional running career was not lack of desire, but being unable to keep myself healthy enough to run, recover, repeat at a world-class level of training. I kept getting interruptions that would not allow me to improve.

If only Dan Frey had written *The Runner's Guide to a Healthy Core* earlier in my career. Here, Dan has given us as close to a secret or shortcut as we can possibly ask for as runners. I wish I had had this book at my disposal when I was at the peak of my running because this book is a how-to guide on keeping yourself healthy and staying on the run-recover-repeat cycle. Dan does an amazing job of speaking in easy-to-understand terms throughout the book and making sense of an otherwise confusing topic, the human body.

This book does a great job of not only laying out how the body functions during running, but diving into how to identify weaknesses before they can become an issue. The strength exercises contained in this book are the best you will find to address each respective issue. What took me years to assemble from other world-class athletes and coaches is available here at your fingertips.

Dan also gives great advice on optimal running form, teaching you the proper posture for breathing and efficient running. These little tips will help knock a lot of seconds off of your times and keep you healthier than you have ever been. I certainly plan to have a copy of this book on hand for my team, if not to make it mandatory reading at the beginning of the year.

Enjoy the book, and here's to many consistent days of training ahead!

—Chris Solinsky,
former US record holder for 10,000 meters

Preface

Running is more popular than ever in the United States. According to the National Sporting Goods Association, more then nine million Americans run 110 or more days per year. Another nineteen million run between twenty-five and 109 days per year. These numbers have continued to climb annually in recent years, as more people recognize how convenient, effective, and rewarding a regular running program can be.

Unfortunately, many of these runners will get injured. Depending on what study you believe, every year anywhere from 25 percent to 80 percent of runners suffer an injury that's significant enough to cut into the quantity and/or quality of their training.

There are many reasons that runners get injured, but underlying almost all of them is asking the body to take on more repetitive strain than it's currently capable of handling. This idea is perhaps easy to accept if you picture a new runner who is overweight and has been sedentary for years. Such a person, you might say, is running to get fit, but doesn't have a body that's yet fit to run. Their excess weight places more stress on their joints when they run, and their years of inactivity will likely mean they lack the general strength to hold good form when they run.

What might not be as easy to accept is that longtime runners, even the fittest and leanest, may be just as susceptible to injury, and for a similar reason—they don't have the strength to maintain good mechanics throughout their runs. The faster and longer they run, the more likely it is that their form will falter, and the more likely it is that they'll eventually develop an injury.

The Core of the Matter

Most runners don't have adequate control of their core musculature. In my practice as a physical therapist, I see it again and again when working with runners—there is weakness somewhere between the abs and hips that sets someone up for an injury in any number of places in the body.

The lack of a strong, healthy core is often made worse by two aspects of modern life. First, many runners spend most of their non-running hours sitting, whether in front of a computer or in a car. Doing so can lead to weakness and postural habits that affect how they run. Second, people feel ever busier. It's common to throw on our running shoes and head out the door without an adequate warm-up, and then after the run to almost instantly get back to the rest of our lives. We don't necessarily consider exercises that build a better running body to be an integral part of a running program.

The fact of the matter is simple: healthy running is deeply rooted in a strong, stable core. In this book, we'll dive deep into what your core truly is. (It's a lot more than having six-pack abs.) We'll see how your core functions when you run. This understanding will show you how essential a healthy core is to your running.

After learning about the runner's core in general, we'll focus on your core specifically. You'll learn how to assess your core for areas of both strength and, even more important, weakness. These weaknesses will become some of the highlights of your fundamental conditioning in the future.

We'll also cover flexibility and soft-tissue mobility in detail, along with a progression of hip strengthening and core stabilization. Finally, we'll look in depth at the relationship between your core and more efficient running mechanics. You'll learn why working to improve your form is as at least as important in running as it is in sports such as skiing or golf, in which people accept the benefits of focusing on technique.

With a good understanding in these areas, you'll be able to design a core program specific to your needs to make you a better runner.

About the Author

I understand running well, but more importantly, I get runners because I've been one almost all of my life. At the suggestion of my physical education teacher, I ran my first road race, a one-mile race held on the city streets of the small Pennsylvania city where I grew up, when I was in third grade. I remember this race well. After lining up in basketball sneakers, I was the odd man out. Luckily, I finished better than I looked with a sub-6:00 mile.

More importantly, I caught the running bug. I continued to run and race throughout high school and went on to compete at the Division I level in cross country and indoor and outdoor track at the University of Delaware. Some of my best times there were 4:05 for 1500 meters and 26:37 for an 8-kilometer cross country course. Since college, I've competed on the track, trails, and roads at distances up to the ultramarathon. I've also run pushing not one, but both of my amazing sons in a stroller, along with two dogs by my side. Some of these runs were crazy, but you do what you have to do to get out. Aside from competition, running is a staple in my life to manage everyday stress and maintain positive energy. Needless to say, I love running.

I knew from a young age that I wanted to be able to apply my love of running to my career. I first studied exercise physiology, and double-minored in strength and conditioning and biology at the University of Delaware. I then earned my Doctor of Physical Therapy degree from the University of New England, in Portland, Maine. I now live and work in the Portland area and am lucky to be in such an active place, as I get to work with runners every day in my practice.

Take some time and digest what you learn about your core as you read this book. My challenge to you: apply one piece of what you read here to every run that you go on. As a runner, you know how small gains can build over time to produce great results. Change is not easy but is often necessary to refine movement. With a good understanding of your core and a well-rounded plan in place, you'll be able to run more efficiently and with less risk for injury.

Chapter 1

What Is the Core?

If I were to ask you what the core of an apple is, what would you say? If you are like most people, then you'd respond that it's the middle of the apple—the part that has the seeds, stem, and the pieces you don't eat. Your answer would likely identify multiple components.

But if I were to ask you what the core of your body is, you might well answer "my abs."

It's true that your abs (short for rectus abdominis) are a significant component of your core. However, if we think about your body as an apple, it makes sense that there should be stuff on the bottom, or the base, of the apple; something in the middle, like the seeds; and something on the top, the stem.

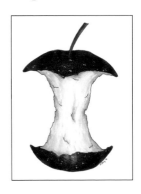

In other words, the core is everything in the middle of your body. Instead of just a good-looking set of six-pack abs, the core is a complex part of your anatomy that is centered in the middle of your body. It's essential that you understand the basic anatomy, bones, and soft tissue that make up your core so that you can better understand how this relates to running. With this knowledge, you will gain a better understanding of proper technique as it relates to conditioning as well as running mechanics, and how to improve both.

Another Way to Visualize the Core

To understand your core in more detail, picture a box of running shoes. The anatomy of this is fairly simple: two sides, a front and a back, a bottom, a top (often connected with a hinge) and, of course, the shoes inside of the box. (One thing missing from this description is the air the inside the box. In Chapter 6, we'll look in depth at why air and, by extension, breathing is such a vital component to core health and performance.)

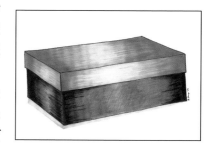

First, picture the bones that make up your core. There's the pelvic girdle, which is made up of two large bones on the side connected through a wedge-shaped sacrum on the back. Extending north off of the sacrum is a series of bones known as vertebrae. There are five in the lumbar section, or lower back, and twelve in the thoracic spine, which is where the ribs originate. The vertebrae articulate through facet joints on the back portion of the bone. There are two joints on the upper-back portion of this and two joints on the lower-back portion.

Between the larger components of each vertebra is an intervertebral disc. This disc is similar to a jelly donut. On the outer portion there's a fibrous, dough-like portion, and on the inside is a jelly-like substance. The ribs wrap around to the front of the body to connect to the chest bone or sternum. Collectively, the thoracic spine, ribs, and sternum are known as the thorax.

For our purpose here, I will also mention the femurs, which are the large thigh bones. These attach to each half of the pelvis through a ball-and-socket joint.

That covers the bones of your core. Now we need to examine the more complex soft-tissue anatomy that binds this all together.

Soft Tissue of the Core

Let's revisit the shoebox analogy and relate this to the softer tissues that make up the core. We'll start with the area that people are most familiar with, the front of the box. As we relate the front of the box to the human core, it's made up of the abdominal wall.

The abdominal wall has multiple layers that overlap throughout your core. The rectus abdominis, or what you see in the famous six-pack abs, is the primary layer in the front. It extends from the sternum to the pubic bones. An isolated contraction of the rectus abdominis would cause your body to hinge forward, as in a sit-up.

We should also make note of the front of the hips as part of the front side of the box. The main group of muscles found here is the iliopsoas, which are more commonly called the hip flexors. This is a group of three muscles that originate off the lumbar spine and back of the pelvis and extend forward of the hip to attach on the upper inside portion of the femur. A contraction of your iliopsoas would either flex your hip, raising your knee off the ground, or pull your spine forward, similar to a sit-up.

Because the hips are an integral piece of the core, let's further examine the other muscles attaching to the pelvis. Just outside of the iliopsoas group lies the tensor fascia latae, or TFL for short. This is a small muscle that attaches to the front of the pelvis, just below the little point that you feel on your hip. It extends into a long, thin tendonous band known as the iliotibial band, which most runners think of only in terms of injury. It runs the length of the outer thigh and attaches just below the knee. The IT band serves to move the thigh outward from the body.

As we move to the inside of the TFL, one of the four quadriceps muscles, called the rectus femoris, is found. We will highlight this muscle because it is the only quadriceps muscle that crosses the hip and attaches on the pelvis. The rectus femoris runs from the front of the hip and extends down to the knee, attaching through the knee cap (patella) to tendon and then eventually to one of the shin bones, the tibia. Like many muscles, it has a dual function; in this case, it's to flex the hip or to extend the knee.

Finally, there are a few muscles on the inner portion of the front of the hip to mention. These muscles originate off of the pubic bones, which is where the pelvis adjoins in the front. First is the adductor group, which is comprised of the adductor magnus, adductor minimus, and adductor longus. These three work together to pull the thigh inward and also help to extend the thigh behind. Two other muscles, the pectineus and the gracilis, have a similar function. They also originate off of the pubic bone and the part of the bone just behind this, and then attach on the thigh. As you can see, the front of the core is quite complex.

Base of the Core

Now let's look at the base of the shoebox. This area is mostly bony, made up by the pelvic girdle. This group of bones resembles a bowl with a big hole in the middle. It's important here to note the pelvic floor, a patchwork of multiple smaller muscles that covers this opening in the pelvis. These muscles are essential in controlling bowel and bladder functions as well as maintaining support for the visceral organs that lie above.

Looking at the sides of the shoebox, we come back to the abdominal wall. Earlier we saw the abdominal wall has layers; these layers are more abundant here than in the front of the core. There are three muscles to consider here. The innermost is the transversus abdominis, or TA; the middle is known as the internal oblique; and the outermost is the external oblique.

The TA can be best visualized as a human back belt. It extends from the lumbar spine, wraps around the sides of the abdomen and connects in the front. When the TA contracts, it compresses circumferentially inward. The obliques have a similar path to the TA but differ in that their fibers overlap in a crisscrossing fashion. They are primarily known to rotate the midsection in a twisting fashion.

Just as we explored the front of the hips in relation to the front of the box, let's look at the outer hips in relation to the sides of the box. The muscles that are acting here originate from the pelvis as well as the sacrum. This area starts to blend closely with the back of the box; for ease of understanding we'll consider them part of the sides. The deepest layer is put together by the hip rotators. These are the piriformis, two obturator muscles, two gemellus muscles, and the quadratus femoris. These muscles contract to rotate the hip in and out.

Then we come to what most people call the glutes, short for gluteal muscles. There are three of these muscles, two found more laterally, the gluteus medius and gluteus minimus. Their primary action is to abduct (move the leg outward from the body). The third, gluteus maximus, arises more from the inner pelvis and sacrum. It's much larger than the other two gluteals—given its size, one of my professors used to call this muscle the London broil of the human. Its massiveness and location give it the action of hip extension, or raising your leg behind you.

Below the glutes are the hamstrings. This is also a group of three muscles: biceps femoris, semimembranosus, and semitendinosus. These all begin on the bone that we sit on, the ischial tuberosity. These powerful muscles run from the sit bone and then attach down below the knee. When they contract, they flex the knee and can extend the thigh.

Back of the Core

Continuing our shoebox analogy, the back of the box will be the location from the top of the pelvis up to the ribs or the lower back. Centrally, we have the lumbar spine. Running along this stack of vertebrae is a group of deeper lower-back muscles known as the rotators and multifidus. These muscles play a small role in rotating and extending the spine or leaning backwards, and ultimately aid in postural control. They are rich in proprioceptors, the feedback sensors that relay information to the brain on the position of a joint, muscle length, or muscle tension. This feedback is essential to your body knowing which position the spine is in. The second, more superficial, larger group of lower-back muscles is known as the erector spinae. These are long bands of muscle that run from the sacrum to the vertebrae and ribs; they act to extend the spine. To round out the deeper lower-back muscles, we have the quadratus lumborum, or QL. Each of the QL lies on either side of the lower back, connecting the lower ribs to the top of the pelvis. When isolated, they help you bend to the side.

Expanding our view of the lower back, we come to one that is likely more recognizable, the latissimus dorsi, or lats for short. The lats are an expansive muscle group extending from the arm to the middle and lower spine, covering most of your back along the way. Their primary function is to pull the arms in to the side from a forward or sideways position.

The lumbar spine can be quite complex and challenging to understand. I often describe it to my patients as one of those high antennas that you see in the distance while driving. Imagine that you were going to make one out of a child's building blocks. You could stack up all of the blocks and go relatively high. In this case, the blocks are the vertebrae in the back.

The challenge, however, is keeping the stack erect—the higher you get, the more unstable it becomes. Choosing a firm base to set your first block on and also aligning the blocks well is essential to make things easier as you go. If you were to add support wires to each block, you would likely be able to make the antenna even higher. In this analogy, these support wires are the muscles of the lower back. When the alignment of all of these is optimal, the lumbar region is more efficient. This will be important to keep in mind when we explore injuries in this area.

Top of the Core

Finally, there's the top of the box. I will mention only one muscle here, the diaphragm. You've probably heard of the diaphragm, but may not have not thought of it as a muscle. After all, you don't walk into the gym and hop on a machine with the goal of strengthening the diaphragm. Instead, it's something you use day in and day out, without really thinking about it, as your primary means of respiration.

But how well are you using it? We'll dive deep into this important answer later. For now, think of this muscle as a large, dome-shaped parachute that covers the roof of your abdominal wall. It acts as a divider between your thoracic cavity, where your heart and lungs are found, and your abdominal cavity. This parachute attaches circumferentially through your sternum, ribs, spine, and some of the other softer tissues that make up your internal abdominal wall. When your diaphragm contracts, it flattens, changing the pressures of your internal cavities and mechanically driving respiration.

Inside the Core

Now we have completed all of the walls of our box: the abs and hips in the front, the pelvic floor on the bottom, the glutes and obliques on the side, the complex lower back on the back, and the diaphragm on the top. To round out our shoebox, we need to look inside.

In this case, the inside of the shoebox is the abdominal cavity. It contains many vital organs, including the kidneys, liver, stomach, intestine, spleen, pancreas, and gall bladder. These organs are, of course, important, but for our purposes we will highlight the space itself on the inside of the box and the air that it contains. This air pressure is essential in maintaining an optimal core.

Make special note of the lumbar and sacral nerves that originate from the lumbar spine. These are the nerves that feed your

legs with the essential electricity that allows your muscles to oper-
ate. These nerves are often compromised from dysfunctions as they
relate to the core, leading to injuries that present elsewhere in the
lower extremities.

It's important to remember that all of the muscles we've examined have multiple actions. For our purposes at this point, we've
been looking at their primary isolated action, meaning what they
do if they contract by themselves. These muscles also have second-
ary or even tertiary actions. Some have a different action if they are
in a different position. Almost all of them have a powerful stabilization component. This purpose is especially important for optimal
running form.

Now that you have a good idea about what the core is, let's look
in depth at why this knowledge is important for you as a runner. In
the next chapter, we'll see how the core works when you run, and
how weakness, tightness, and instability in the core can make you
slower and more susceptible to injury.

Chapter 2

Why Is the Core Important for Runners?

Your body's movement and your running gait are strongly influenced by the control of your core. Biomechanics, or how the structure of the body relates to movement, suggests that your core does not always function in isolation but has a close connection to how the other parts of your body function too.

Do you recall singing the "Dem Bones" song when you were growing up? It's the song that says the leg bone is connected to the knee bone, the knee bone is connected to the thigh bone, the thigh bone is connected to the back bone, and so on. Thinking about this song as we approach your body's biomechanics will help you appreciate the core's connection to the rest of our body.

The point is that the body operates as an extensive chain. The core is a large and powerful link, but without the other smaller links such as legs or arms, the chain is not complete. A weak link could be anywhere in the chain and may affect that area, another area, or both. An example of this is that stubborn pebble that finds its way into your running shoe. You are still able to run with it in your shoe but you may find it uncomfortable. You can stop and remove it, or keep running and alter your gait. By changing your gait, the foot no longer hurts but you start to notice that your back is bothering you because of the change in your mechanics. This is often the beginning of an injury and makes understanding the mechanics of your body crucial for injury prevention.

The Running Gait Cycle

A running gait cycle is the time it takes for one foot to contact the ground, leave the ground, and then contact again. It takes about a half- to three-quarters of a second for most runners, but as fast as it is, a lot of things happen during that time. To better understand your core function during running, we will break the running gait cycle into eight phases. These eight phases will be further broken down into stance (when the foot is in contact with the ground) or swing (when the foot is in the air).

Stance Phases:

Initial Contact (IC)
Loading Response (LR)
Mid Stance (MS)
Terminal Stance (TS)

Swing Phases:

Pre-Swing (PSw)
Initial Swing (ISw)
Mid-Swing (Sw)
Terminal Swing (TSw)

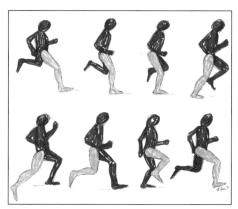

The eight phases of the running gait cycle: IC, LR, MS, TS, PSw, ISw, Sw, TSw.

Initial Contact: The foot has a variety of ways to contact the ground: heel strike, mid-foot strike, and forefoot strike. Your foot can also land more toward the inside, outside, or middle portion of the foot. This begins the first phase of gait, or IC.

Research suggests that how your foot strikes may not be as important as where your foot strikes. If IC occurs closer to your body or underneath, rather than too far out in front, the contact force is absorbed better. When your foot lands closer to you, you will likely have less of a heel strike pattern and your knee will be slightly more flexed, creating more of a spring in your body. Picture someone jumping up and down. If you jump with your knees locked straight, your landing will be more firm. If you allow your knees to flex when you

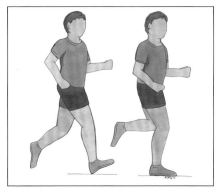

Landing position when running: excessive reach in front of the body (left) and appropriate landing closer to the body (right).

land, it will be softer. The softer landing minimizes bone and joint stress.

Because IC represents the first time the foot contacts the ground during a gait cycle, your core needs to prepare the body for a load. The position of the pelvis, lumbar spine, and thorax is crucial here. If this alignment is not correct, then the muscles will not function at an optimal level. The spine from a lateral view should have a double "S" curvature without an excessive curvature in the lumbar, thoracic, or cervical region. Your pelvis should be relatively flat from front to back. One of the most common problems in this area is an increased forward lumbar curvature and a pelvis that is excessively tilted forward. The combination of these creates poor body stabilization.

The two primary muscles that act in this phase are the gluteus

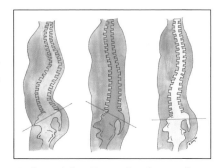

Left to right: Excessive forward pelvic tilt with increased lumbar extension. Excessive backward pelvic tilt with increased lumbar flexion. Neutral hip and lumbar spine alignment.

maximus and the adductor magnus. They help stabilize the femur (large thigh bone) in preparation for landing. Appropriate alignment here will make stability easier in the later phases.

Loading Response: From IC we transition to the LR of your gait. You can also think of this phase as the absorption phase. Your body has to accept the impulse from the foot contacting the ground. This is done through the softer tissues in addition to your bones and joints. By dispersing the initial impulse throughout various structures making up the chain, the isolated segments are not loaded as much. This minimizes stress, thereby helping to decrease your risk of injury.

The core's function during this phase is described with one word: stiffness. The core must prepare rapidly for the external load from the contact with the ground. To do that, it braces forcefully. The tighter it becomes, the more it is able to stabilize your spine and pelvis in a neutral position.

For example, if you were going to get hit in the stomach, what would you do? You would instinctually brace your abdomen. This creates a stiff abdominal wall of armor to protect you. The tighter you become, the more you are able to sustain the blow. This is similar to landing on the ground when running. This stiffness minimizes extraneous movement, such as a drop of your pelvis from side to side or a collapse of your knee inward. Both of these motions happen predominantly in the frontal plane.

It is important to understand the three planes of the body to focus on what we are trying to achieve through exercise and mechanics work. The three planes are known as the frontal, sagittal, and transverse.

Frontal Plane: The frontal plane divides the front and the back. It goes across your body through your arm, leg, torso, and then passes through the other half of your body.

Sagittal Plane: The sagittal plane runs front to back and divides the body into right and left halves. It goes from the back portion of your body, through your midsection, and then out through your front.

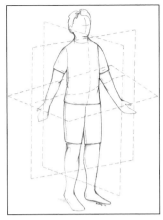

Transverse Plane: Unlike the other two planes, this is horizontal to the ground. It separates the body into top and bottom halves.

Your hip musculature is also important during this phase. The gluteus maximus and adductor magnus are highly

Planes of the body: frontal, sagittal, and transverse.

active. They act in conjunction with the hamstrings to control the amount that the femur flexes forward when landing. The tensor fascia lata, gluteus medius, and gluteus minimus play different roles. They control the pelvis to prevent hip drop, meaning the opposite hip will fall downward if the amount of force when contacting the ground is too excessive for the stability of your core and strength in your

outer hip muscles. Hip drop creates poor lower extremity alignment and increases susceptibility for injury.

Mid-Stance: From LR, your body moves into MS, which represents the time when your body has the most direct connection to the ground. Your foot will be flat and underneath you. This phase is an excellent time to look at the posture that your body holds while you are running.

When you look from the side, you should see a straight alignment.

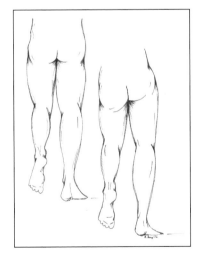

Level hip position (left) and hip drop in right stance (right).

It should be easy to draw a line from the foot on the ground through the hip, shoulder, and ears. Notice I said straight posture and not vertical. Rather than being vertical, you should have a slight lean forward during your stride. This lean should occur through a hinge at your ankle and not a hinge in your core. If you hinge from the hips or lumbar spine, you lose stability, decreasing overall control and increasing your risk for injury.

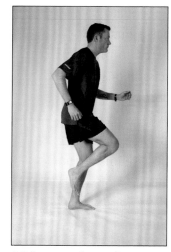

Mid-stance phase of running.

The vertical position can alter the mechanics of your core. The hips are too far behind and the stomach is sticking excessively forward. The effect of this faulty position trickles up the chain, causing the lower ribs to protrude forward. Picture a pair of scissors with the top being your lower rib cage and the bottom being the top of your pelvis. When they are too far open, it creates inefficient posture by making someone look like they have a sway back posture with the stomach protruding towards the front.

Core muscle function during MS initiates the extension of the femur behind you, as well as preventing the pelvis from dropping. Gluteus maximus is a powerful extender of your hip. It should initiate more of this motion than your hamstring, which should fire less during this phase. Hamstring dominance is common for runners. This is the phase of the gait cycle in which it begins to be a problem.

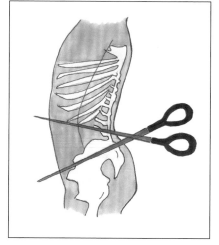

Open scissors posture.

The well-developed and appropriately firing gluteus maximus has a better line of pull to perform the extension of the hip compared to the hamstring. A poor forward tilt of the pelvis or open-scissor position will hinder the gluteals, causing more hamstring dominance. This sets them up for overuse. They are not able to extend the hip as well as the glute, which makes them overwork, and they will be more important in an upcoming phase of your gait. If the hamstrings expend their energy now, they will remain active during more of the gait cycle than necessary.

As they do in LR, the gluteus medius and minimus, along with TFL, continue to work collectively to control the pelvis in the front plane. They do, however, begin to function less at this point, as some of the larger muscles begin to take over.

Terminal Stance: Moving from MS to TS the leg passes underneath the body and extends out behind. The body is at the point where it begins to roll off the forefoot into a push-off position. TS can be thought of as the propulsion phase of gait. It will also represent the last stance phase before the foot leaves the ground.

TS is when you will see triple extension in the body. This term is common in the world of strength and conditioning due to its importance in maximizing power when pushing off the ground in running, jumping, or pushing activities. Triple extension occurs when you have maximal extension through the hip, knee, and ankle. This position recruits gluteus maximus at the hip but also a number of other large and powerful muscles needed for performance.

Here's a simple way to better understand triple extension. Stand up and try the following two jumps and you will feel the difference in power:

Partial Two Leg Jump: Start in a squat position. Jump upward, reaching for the sky, but do not allow your knees to straighten fully. You will notice your hips stay a little bent as well. Allow your knees to bend when landing.

Full Two Leg Jump: Start in the same squat position. Jump up as high as you're able, again reaching for the sky, but this time allow your knees to straighten out. You will notice that your hips also straighten and your toes will probably point more toward the ground.

You should notice that in the second jump you are able to go higher, and the jump probably feels more natural and explosive. This is triple extension.

The core remains active in stabilizing the hips and spine here. Iliopsoas, rectus femoris, and TFL flexibility are extremely important at this point. If these are restricted they will limit the ability of the femur to extend behind the body adequately. This limitation is common in runners and leads to multiple compensations throughout the body.

The first compensation is an overextension of the lumbar spine. The iliopsoas group attaches not only to the hip but extends higher up to the lumbar spine. If the length of these is too short, they will pull the lumbar spine and pelvis forward in an effort to lengthen. This constant tugging can create problems.

The second compensation is an over-rotation of the trunk. TS represents a time during your gait when you will see the most transverse plane rotation through your trunk. The torso and hips will rotate in opposite directions. Although this is normal, the degree to which it occurs needs to be well-controlled. Limited flexibility in the front of the hip will create more of this rotation, causing excessive twisting through your spine. This twisting will further pull your pelvis and spine from an optimal position to stabilize.

Pre-Swing: PSw is the first phase of the gait cycle where you find the lower extremity leaving the ground. The leg is still behind you but the knee is flexed and the extremity is beginning to move forward.

Iliopsoas and your adductor group, specifically adductor magnus and gracilis, initiate the flexing of your thigh in the forward direction. Rectus femoris also aids in this. It is important that these muscles do the work, to allow your hamstring to be less active. They see some action in flexing the knee at this point, but should not be the primary workhorses. Runners who tend to over-recruit the hamstrings tend to have a high heel rise—or butt kick—behind them.

Try the "Dirty Shirt Test." The next time you go out for a run after it rains, check your shirt afterward. How much dirt did you kick up your back? When we see the dirt line all over the back of the shirt—and maybe even extending to your head—it is likely that your heel is traveling too high. This needs to be controlled to minimize hamstring load. Your hamstrings will be heavily loaded in the final two phases of gait.

Initial Swing: ISw is an extension of PSw, but now the foot has entirely left the ground and is moving forward. Some call this the "acceleration phase" of swing, which is a better visual. The lower extremity is lifted off the ground and picks up speed as it travels to a point underneath the torso. The iliopsoas is highly active in this process. It not only pulls the thigh forward but is also essential in making sure that the foot clears the ground as it travels forward. The inner thigh, including the adductor longus and gracilis, also continues to remain active, helping to pull the femur forward.

Mid-Swing: After the thigh has accelerated forward maximally, you will be in MSw. MSw will look similar to the MS phase, as described earlier, but on opposite legs. This means that the MSw leg will have maximal hip flexion with the knee elevated off the ground. The foot will be under the torso, but moving forward. This is a transition phase of your gait for this leg. We know that in ISw the leg is accelerating forward; we will soon find out that during TSw the leg needs to decelerate. MSw is where this change of momentum will occur.

Your driving muscles through the front and inner hip begin to quiet as the back portion of the thigh and hip takes over. The hamstrings begin to fire strongly to slow the lower leg from moving too far forward. If the hamstrings are in the wrong position and not well-controlled, the potential for injury is high.

To better understand this, look at a baseball pitcher. It can be exciting to see how fast a pitcher can throw the ball: Was it ninety or even 100-plus miles per hour? If you decided you wanted to be a successful pitcher, you would probably work diligently on the muscles that throw the ball with a lot of force. For the most part, these lie on the front of the body. The average person would probably not be able to throw 100 miles per hour, but could probably throw with more velocity after training. However, we need to be able to balance this out. If your arm is throwing with more force, you need to have better control at the shoulder and especially the backside of your arm and shoulder to slow down the arm. Without this essential balance, the muscles on the back of the body strain to control the amount of force that was created in moving the ball forward. The repetitive stress of this leads to injury.

This is similar to the hamstring. Many runners think of running fast and pushing hard, but don't think about how well they can control this. Monster quadriceps are developed, but without sufficient hamstrings to balance them out. This creates dominance through the front of the leg without the balance in the back of the leg to adequately slow down the leg. This causes repetitive excessive stress on the hamstring and may lead to injury.

Now, imagine yourself as the baseball pitcher again. You have trained for months to throw as hard as you can and have maxed out your velocity. What would you do next? We have bypassed one of the most important aspects of movement: the mechanics. By taking this hard-throwing pitcher and cleaning up his or her mechanics, a higher velocity would likely result. This would include stability around the core and hips, along with better control in the legs, trunk, and arm.

These mechanics are just as important in running. The hamstrings attach to the bone that we sit on. If this bone is elevated and farther back than it should be, such as in the open scissor position, the hamstring has excessive length and does not function at its best. Even if this hamstring is strong, the position alone could put it in a disadvantageous position.

Our core is important in controlling the hip and trunk dissociation that was mentioned earlier. The legs and arms are moving in an opposite fashion. This rapid change in force is countered through the stability of the core. As you move through the MSw on one side and MS on the other side of your body's phases of gait, this core control is necessary. Here is where the arms cross from front to back, as well as the legs. Along with this, the hips and trunks will cross paths as they begin to rotate in the opposite direction. The same deceleration of your hamstring is necessary in your core muscles to minimize the amount that the spine rotates in the transverse plane.

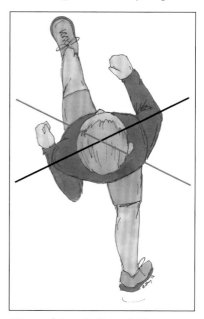

Terminal Swing: In this final phase, the leg in the air is moving into its maximal range in front of the body. It is preparing the location in which the foot will contact the ground and also the posture that the body will take when this occurs. Just as the ISw is the acceleration phase of swing, this is the deceleration phase of swing.

The hamstrings are also highly active in TSw. There is an increase

Hip and trunk dissociation while running. Notice opposite relationship of shoulders (black line) and pelvis (blue line).

in gluteal and adductor action as well. These muscles work hard to decelerate the leg from moving forward. Better control will allow the leg to contact the ground in a more ideal position, with the knee slightly flexed rather than excessively extended. If it does overextend, it will stress the hamstrings more and increase the amount of load that the bones and joints in the lower extremity will need to absorb.

The gluteus medius, gluteus minimus, and TFL all begin to fire here. They work together to stabilize in preparation to accept the load. The rapid pre-activation of these, along with the rest of the core, helps to brace the midsection. This firm stabilization sets up an ideal foundation for the transition back to the first phase of your gait, IC.

The Importance of Your Upper Extremities

It is important that you do not forget arm swing. Arm swing can be either a driving force of your mechanics or a result of your mechanics. It is important to recognize that your lower extremities and upper extremities, in the end, are going to work together. They act in direct opposition of one another to create balance. The left arm drives forward as the right leg moves backward and so on. This counter force from upper to lower is transferred through your core.

We will talk later about exercises and drills to control your arm swing. Because we have just gone over trunk and hip dissociation, it is a good time to mention how arm swing can be a result of mechanics.

Take, for example, a runner with poor flexibility through the front of her hips. This creates excessive pelvis rotation and forward tilt. A similar demonstration of this could occur in a runner who has appropriate flexibility here but lacks the stability to control her core. One way or another, she has increased trunk rotation. Due to this over-rotation of the trunk, the arms swing moderately across the body. This runner could correct her arm swing, but this faulty mechanic is actually derived from the hips and core.

It is important to recognize that a number of other muscles fire during your gait cycle. The motion and torque at the knee and ankle play a crucial role in your gait. We are focusing on the proximal hip and core musculature, but all of the links in the body's chain have a key role in your gait.

Remember that when running, all eight phases will take place in less than a second. Due to the rapid nature of this sport, the foundations of movement, including mechanics, strength, flexibility, mobility, and stability, are important. A poor foundation of conditioning and mechanics can lead to an inefficient gait and injury.

Chapter 3

Injuries to the Core

A high school cross country runner begins to have lower back pain while running. For the first week or two, the pain is mild and present only with higher-intensity workouts. In the second to third week, the pain increases and begins to linger after running, usually lasting through most of that day. It is gone by the next day. The athlete goes to his primary care doctor, who recommends rest for a few days and regular icing. After a few days of diligent ice and rest, the athlete returns to practice. The pain returns immediately. A follow-up phone call to the primary care doctor initiates a referral to an orthopedic physician.

The orthopedist provides flexibility exercises, including hamstring, hip, and lower-back stretching. He also recommends further rest, ice, and routine over-the-counter anti-inflammatory medication. After a week of this regimen, the pain is still present at low levels without running. The physician orders an X-ray of the lumbar spine, which shows two questionable areas. The athlete is referred for further imaging, which reveals two clear lumbar stress fractures. These fractures are on both sides of the vertebrae on a small bony area called the pars interarticularis. The patient is told to continue rest, ice, anti-inflammatory medicine, and is prescribed a back brace to be worn as much as possible.

After many weeks, the athlete returns to running and is able to progress back to running and racing in the brace. Gradually he phases out of the brace, but a dull pain in the lower back is present at times. This persists off and on for the next few years.

During his senior year, coaches recommended weight lifting and core strengthening. As the runner begins this, he notices that any time he does motions that involve a lot of back extension or bending backward, his back is uncomfortable. In contrast, when he does a sit-up, it feels better. He begins doing regular core exercises that feel good for the back. The athlete returns to train and compete without discomfort in college and later life.

The athlete is me. This experience, as frustrating as it was, sparked my interest in sports medicine. Today, patients come to me daily with similar stories. I can relate well to their struggles and their desire to return to running as soon as possible.

Much of the missing link in stories like this is education. Runners tend to know their bodies well and paint a picture of their injuries through their words before I begin to examine them. I would love for my patients to catch the injury before it turns into something more. If it does become full-blown, I want them to be able to treat it appropriately. This chapter, along with the next, will help in this area.

Background on Injuries

Injuries are frustrating for everyone. Running injuries are even more frustrating. Think of fellow runners on your team or in your running group. They are determined, motivated, and goal-driven. Whether trying to lose weight, control life stressors, finish a 5K, or set a personal record, they have a motive and do not want any roadblocks along the way. If a small twinge or soreness begins, runners tend to brush it aside as long as they can continue to run. Unfortunately, these lesser symptoms tend to be precursors for larger injuries.

The second factor is the nature of most running injuries. They tend to start slowly and are long in the making. This chronic nature is different from an acute injury. Someone who rolls an ankle while playing football goes from healthy to hurt in a matter of seconds and can describe exactly what happened and when. A chronic injury usually dates back weeks, months, or even years. A runner will be able to explain what hurts and how far into a run it starts, but when the pain began is usually blurry. A chronic presentation often needs short-term treatment to calm down the pain, as well as a longer-term plan to reeducate movement or mechanics so that the true underlying problem can be addressed. This is much more involved than rehabbing an ankle sprain, which usually takes a month.

As we talk about acute versus chronic injuries, it is important to understand the word "tendonitis" better. This is a word that is often misused by runners. By definition, "tendonitis" means "acute tendon injury accompanied by inflammation." Tendonitis is more acute in nature and should be easy to calm down with rest, soft-tissue mobility and flexibility, ice, and possibly oral anti-inflammatories.

If tendonitis is present for a longer period of time it often evolves into tendonosis. The definition of "tendonosis" is a chronic tendon injury with degeneration at the cellular level and no inflammation. The key to this definition is that it does not involve inflammation; therefore, if tendonosis is treated with the same prescription as tendonitis, you will likely not see any improvement in your symptoms. This will often need to be treated with more extensive exercises and may require a more in-depth examination by a professional to determine underlying causes of the pathology.

The final word to keep in mind is "tendinopathy," which is more of a catch-all meaning "disease of a tendon." Tendinopathy is a better word choice if the true diagnosis is unknown.

Core injuries, excluding the hips, are not as common in runners when compared to injuries of the knees, ankles, and feet. However, the injuries that do present in the hips and core tend to be stubborn. They are often more chronic in nature and typically have a direct relationship to gait and running mechanics. Let's go through running injuries found in the core. We'll start with bone and joint injuries.

Lower Back Pain (Bone and Joint)

Cause

Lower back pain may stem from deeper structures than the muscles, arising from the bones and joints of the spine. The facet joints of the spine or the vertebral junctions at the disc can become inflamed from excessive load. This load can be caused by multiple factors. Some are running-related, such as excessive impact or poor mechanics. It may also be caused by lifestyle factors that are smaller in nature but cumulatively overload the spine, such as poor posture during daily sitting or bending. Poor core alignment may also lead to this type of pain.

Diagnoses such as osteoarthrosis or osteoarthritis, degenerative disc disease, or degenerative joint disease may be underlying factors for this type of lower back pain.

Presentation

Bone-derived lower back pain is likely duller initially and can be present during all times of the day. It may be exacerbated when running, but might feel better with movement. The pain is too deep to palpate and usually hard to localize to just one spot. It is important to recognize that the softer tissues may often be affected simultaneously. They may spasm to protect the spine.

Self-Treatment

Initial treatment should include rest from running to decrease impact on the spine, along with light lower back and hip stretching. Lifestyle changes are often an important consideration. Examine day-to-day postures and try modifications to your work position, such as standing instead of sitting. Also consider your driving posture and altering your sleeping positions. In the long term, you will likely benefit from core strengthening and stability exercises.

When to Seek Help

This type of pain is more common in runners who are in their thirties or older. Runners who are younger than this should seek medical attention if the pain has lasted more than five to seven days and conservative treatment has failed. Given the complexity of this type of pain, it is important to have an appropriate diagnosis to best treat the cause and symptoms. For runners who are middle-aged or older, or have been having progressive and longer-lasting symptoms, seek medical attention before continuing activity to properly diagnose the origin of the pain. Anyone having lower back pain that is accompanied by numbness, tingling, burning, or pain going into one or both legs needs to seek medical attention promptly. These are indicators of nerve involvement.

Osteoarthritis/Osteoarthrosis (Hip or Spine)

Cause

Osteoarthritis and osteoarthrosis are degenerative in nature over a long time. Osteoarthrosis is degenerative change of a joint. If this joint becomes inflamed, it is known as osteoarthritis or OA. It may be affected by posture, muscular imbalance, and/or mechanics.

Presentation

OA causes pain that comes from the joint itself. It can be present in any joint in the body, but for our purposes, the focus is the ball-and-socket hip joints and the vertebral junctions in the lower back. OA is typically worse with extremes of movement. It is worse with prolonged static positions such as sleeping, sitting, driving, or standing. On the other end of the spectrum, it can be exacerbated by excessive walking or running. It typically feels better with light constant motion, such as a conservative amount of walking or running.

Hip arthritis is characterized by pain that feels deep in the hip and may radiate into the groin. Crunching or grinding sensations may also be felt with movement. Spine arthritis has localized lower back pain that is central over the spine. It is not able to be palpated.

Self-Treatment

There is no cure for osteoarthrosis; however, if it is inflammatory in origin, or OA, it can be managed. Initial treatment should include limiting duration of static activities, as well as prolonged activities. Perform light regular exercise as tolerated. Light hip and spine flexibility may be beneficial. Longer-term core stabilization and postural control are key.

When to Seek Help

If symptoms are lower level (described above), continue conservative management for up to two weeks. If symptoms increase in intensity or do not respond to conservative treatment, it is important that the pain be examined by a professional.

Spondylolysis/Spondylolisthesis

Cause

Spondylolysis and spondylolisthesis have a similar origin, often from repetitive and excessive load to the lumbar spine in an extended or backward bent position. Excessive extension places an increased load on the back part of the vertebra, leading to stress and often fracture of part of the bone. This is called spondylolysis. Spondylolisthesis differs because the vertebra has fractured and then begins to slip forward, or occasionally backward. Runners who have poor hip flexibility or poor core stability often do not control the spine well when running, making them more susceptible.

Presentation

These diagnoses present similarly with pain central in the lumbar spine and most often just above the sacrum. The pain normally increases as the day goes on and with exercise. Most individuals find that the pain is worse when extending the lower back and feels better when flexing the lumbar spine forward, such as touching your toes or sitting in a recliner. These conditions tend to be progressive, meaning that in the early stages there is minimal pain but as the weeks go by, the pain is usually more intense and limiting. The later stages are often accompanied by more diffuse lower-back discomfort and pain, along with muscular spasm. It is more common among youth who are still growing, normally high school age, but can also occur in later years.

Self-Treatment

In the earlier stages, the pain is usually minimal and manageable with light flexibility exercises for the iliopsoas, iliotibial band, and hamstrings. Cross training with non-impact activities is normally tolerated well. Keep a heavy focus on retraining the core to minimize the extension during running. Initially this will entail appropriate core stability training with particular focus on a neutral lumbar pelvis and spine. Later stages will progress to incorporating this focus into daily activities and running.

When to Seek Help

Most individuals do not realize that this is the true pathology in the earlier stages. In the earlier stages, this injury is often perceived as a dull and localized back pain. If the pain is following a progressive pattern—not only increasing during running, but also increasing from run to run—it is essential that it be examined by a professional. A fracture of the spine can be quite serious and needs an appropriate diagnosis to best direct treatment.

Hip Impingement Syndrome

Cause

Hip impingement has become better understood in recent years. Historically, pain in the front of the hip was often diagnosed simply as hip pain. Now medical professionals treat pain there in varying degrees, from conservative rehabilitation to surgical intervention.

Hip impingement can be structural or mechanical. In structural hip impingement, the bone is shaped poorly and does not allow the hip to move well. This can be caused by a pincer lesion, which is a bird beak–like projection off the hip socket, or a cam lesion, which is a rounded projection on the femur. Both of these bony structures can limit the hip's ability to move properly, causing a pinching in

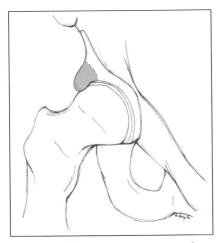

Structural hip impingement with a pincer lesion.

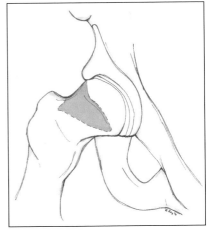

Structural hip impingement with a cam lesion.

the front of the hip. Repetitive pinching leads to inflammation and pain.

Hip impingement can also be mechanical when no structural block is limiting the hip's range of motion. Instead, the hip's movement may be limited by poor positioning and control of the hip and pelvis. Picture the open-scissor position. A pelvis that is tilted excessively forward will also move the hip socket forward. When the femur is raised up during a running stride forward, it can bind in the front of the hip. This binding is the impingement. When running up a hill, the femur needs to be raised higher and often exacerbates the symptoms more.

Presentation

Hip impingement presents with pain most often across the front of the hip that travels into the groin. It feels like deep pain, which tends to increase with physical activities and even more with activities or positions that flex the hip to a deeper range of motion, such as running up a hill, doing high knees, or sitting for prolonged periods of time. Pain is normally less when stretching the front of the hip.

Self-Treatment

Structural and mechanical hip impingements are initially treated similarly. It's important to take a break from running, but non-impact cross training activities that don't require hip-flexed positions are fine. Biking should be performed in a more upright position, and elliptical stride length should be limited. Swimming is often tolerated well. Hip flexibility is important to decrease the load on the front of the hip. Longer-term treatment should focus on core stability and retraining core position during activities to minimize the pelvis falling forward. Individuals who sit a lot should consider a sit/stand workstation to minimize stress on the front of the hip during the day. Also, runners who drive long distances will benefit from seat modifications to open the hip angle while driving.

When to Seek Help

Mechanical hip impingement often responds well to conservative treatment. If symptoms are not improving after three to four weeks of self-treatment, it should be examined by a professional. Structural hip impingement may not respond to conservative treatment and may require further surgical intervention. Hip impingement that has been going on for longer periods of time may cause further degenerative changes in the hip; therefore, it should be assessed by a professional before treatment. Pain that is more acute and intense should also be evaluated by a medical professional to rule out fraying or a tear of the labrum.

Femur or Pelvis Stress Injury

Cause

Stress injuries develop when a bone is unable to tolerate the amount of stress being placed on it. For runners, this is normally a result of overuse. Bone is extremely strong and adaptable, but if stressed too much or too fast it does not have the time to build and handle the applied load. After excessive intensity or repetition, the load will cause inflammation and structural fatigue in the bone. These early stages are known as a stress reaction. I view this as a bruise to the bone—it is damaged, but it has no clear signs of a fracture. If the stress continues to be placed on the bone, it may progress to a stress fracture, and a visible hairline fracture can be seen on an X-ray.

Presentation

A stress injury or stress fracture can present in any bone. They are not as common in the hip or pelvis, but can occur. Runners often get them in neck of the femur. Pain presents across the front of the hip and into the groin. The pain is primarily with activity and increases from run to run. In the beginning phases, the pain is minimal and normally not felt until later in the run. As the injury advances, the pain is more intense and can start from the first step of the run. Symptoms are noticed with impact on the ground. Pain may linger after a run, but normally after a period of rest, the symptoms will resolve. If the bone is more irritated, often with a full-blown stress fracture, pain may be present with standing and walking and may even cause limping. These injuries tend to happen to beginning runners, those who have recently increased training volume or intensity, or runners who have been training at a higher volume for a sustained period of time.

Self-Treatment

Running is an impact sport and there are only so many ways to control this. Two of these are body weight and mechanics. Someone who is overweight will place increased load on their bone when contacting the ground. This, however, is not always the most common person to have a stress injury. Runners who land harder on the ground will cause more stress to their bone. This may be audible during running, like a foot slap or pounding. Work on correcting these problems only after the stress injury has healed.

In addition, appropriate core and lower extremity alignment is essential to more efficient loading of the bone. For example, hip weakness may cause excessive knee collapse inward when running. This motion could go on to stress the bone more than it would if it was well-controlled, setting up a risk for injury.

When to Seek Help

Stress injuries are serious and need to be examined by a medical professional. If this diagnosis is made, often eight or more weeks of rest will be prescribed, followed by a slow and guided progression back to running. During this rest time, professional guidance on strength, core stability, and mechanics retraining is recommended. A running gait assessment is also recommended before a full return to running to assess for mechanics that may be overloading the bone. Finally, it may be important to have bone composition testing and nutrition assessed. These can be underlying variables, especially for runners who have had repeated stress injuries.

Now let's turn to soft-tissue injuries in the back and core.

Lower Back Pain (Soft Tissue in Nature)

Cause

Lower back pain is a generic diagnosis that is often all-encompassing. It may include pain originating from the muscles around the lower back, such as the erector spinae or quadratus lumborum. These are often not strained or torn from running-related injuries, but may stiffen or spasm from guarding or overuse.

One of the most common causes for soft tissue lower back pain is poor core position while running. It may present with the open scissor posture that was described earlier. Tightness through the iliopsoas, TFL, and rectus femoris can lead to excess forward position of the pelvis, causing a shortening of the lower back muscles. Instability of the core muscles may also be a culprit. Poor gluteal, hip, and core strength may lead to excessive rotational motion or a forward pelvis that could cause excessive soft-tissue loading. Running mechanics alone can also lead to this pain. A runner who is over-striding will often have excessive motion in the hips and back that is translated above the pelvis to the lower back.

Presentation

Symptoms of a soft-tissue lower back injury often include pain across the middle to lower back that is tender when palpating the area. The pain is often more diffuse and may arise during or after running. The pain is typically gone by the next day.

Self-Treatment

Initial short-term treatment should include a few days of rest from running. Cross training with non-impact activities should be fine during this time. Flexibility exercises for the iliopsoas, rectus femoris, and lower back should be done if they are able to be performed symptom-free. (We will take a look at these later.) Light intensity and longer, 60-second holds should be maintained. Perform two to three sets, two times a day. Ice or heat may also be used to help control symptoms.

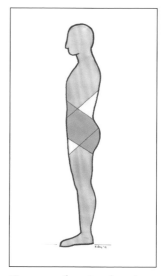

Core quadrants, showing tight front of hips and lower back (light shaded region) and weak abdomen and glutes (dark shaded region).

The importance of treating this longer term often relates to improving the balance of tightness and weakness in your core. Improving this balance is essential to minimize risk and treat lower back pain. Treating this injury in quadrants often makes it easier. Improve gluteal, hip, abdomen, and core strength. Stretch and mobilize the tissue of the lower back and the front of the hips.

When to Seek Help

Soft-tissue pain should heal quickly with conservative treatment, especially if it is from overuse. If symptoms are not improving or getting worse after one week of self-treatment, seek further medical attention. Note that symptoms originating from a mechanical imbalance may take much longer to improve. If symptoms are improving after the first week and not lasting more than twenty-four hours after running, continue to treat conservatively. If symptoms increase or are longer lasting, seek professional help to rule out other injuries and develop a longer-term treatment plan.

Greater Trochanteric Bursitis

Cause

The greater trochanter bursa lies on the outside of the hip. This fluid-filled sac is designed to minimize friction between the bone and the softer tissues that are superficial to it. If excessive load is placed on this bursa it can become inflamed and painful. Often weakness through the outer gluteal muscles and instability in the core may lead to excessive rotation and collapse of the knee inward during running. This creates an increased load on the outer hip and ultimately the bursa. With the repetition that accompanies running, this poor alignment causes increased pressure and friction in the bursa, leading to pain.

Presentation

Pain is present on the outside of the hip at the greater trochanter or the outer hip bone, which is just below the pelvic crest. It is often tender to touch and when putting pressure on it, such as lying on your side. Pain tends to increase with running, but also walking or standing. Symptoms are normally lessened after periods of rest.

Self-Treatment

Initial treatment should include limiting activities that are irritating it, along with ice placed over the tender area to help decrease the inflammation. This treatment often will make it feel better, but rarely treats it in its entirety. Given the underlying mechanical limitations, it is important to develop a comprehensive treatment plan.

This plan should include proximal iliopsoas, TFL, and hip rotator flexibility. Soft-tissue treatment of these areas as well as the IT band will also benefit. This should be viewed as the staple in this program, but not the fix. Long-term focus should be placed on lateral hip strengthening specific to the gluteal muscles. It is also important to emphasize core stability. During strength and stability work, pay attention to the alignment of your lower body, being careful to minimize pronation through your foot and inward collapse of the knee.

When to Seek Help

Conservative treatment is often effective for this condition. With the above treatment plan, an improvement in symptoms should be felt quickly and continue to resolve with time. If pain is not improving in three to four weeks, this should be assessed by a professional to determine the appropriate treatment plan. This diagnosis can be stubborn and therefore consistent, and longer-term compliance to treatment is essential.

Gluteus Medius Tendinopathy/Tendonitis

Cause

Gluteus medius tendinopathy or tendonitis is caused by excessive load to the lower tendon attachment site of this muscle. It often originates from underlying hip weakness and poor biomechanical alignment when running, similar to greater trochanteric bursitis.

Presentation

Pain is found on and just above the greater trochanter or outer hip bone. It may also spread above this area and into the glute in the back. It can often be palpated and is painful to the touch. It is aggravated by activity and normally increases in intensity with duration. Pain will often remain after you stop an activity, but at a lower level.

It often will feel better in one to three days if the aggravating activity has not been performed. Individuals may notice stiffness and a tight feeling in this area first thing in the morning or after sedentary periods of time. This normally improves quickly and there is no pain until the higher level of stress is again introduced.

Self-Treatment

Initial focus should be on rest, ice, and soft-tissue mobility, which in this case involves self-massage using a foam roller, ball, rolling stick, or even your hand. (We will cover this in detail in Chapter 7.) Icing and avoiding activities will decrease symptoms quickly. Soft-tissue mobility to the tendon and muscles around it should help overall healing in the short term. Long-term focus should be placed heavily on lateral hip strengthening and core stability. If it has been going on for a long time, isolated gluteus medius exercises may be beneficial.

When to Seek Help

If symptoms do not respond to the above treatment plan quickly, seek professional medical attention after three to four weeks. In more extreme cases, a rare tear of this tendon may develop. This could require surgical intervention.

Iliopsoas Tendinopathy/Tendonitis

Cause

Iliopsoas tendinopathy or tendonitis is caused by excessive loading of the hip flexor tendon. This is not that common in runners, but may develop from activities that place an increased load on the front of the hip, such as hill training or speed work. An injury pathology with a similar presentation, apophysitis, may be seen in younger individuals who are still developing. This is caused by excessive tugging of the iliopsoas tendon on its attachment to the bone. Repetition of this stress can lead to inflammation and pain.

Presentation

Iliopsoas tendinopathy is characterized by pain in the front of the hip, which may wrap slightly into the groin. This pain can often be palpated but in some instances is hard to localize and described as being "deeper." It follows a similar presentation of the gluteus medius in that symptoms normally increase with activity and improve with rest.

Self-Treatment

Focus on rest and soft-tissue mobility first. You may try ice, but due to the depth of the tissue, it may not be effective. Light hip flexor and quad flexibility exercises should be performed early in treatment. A long-term focus should be on developing strength through the hip flexor and also globally through the hips and core.

When to Seek Help

Most respond quickly to the above approach. If pain is not responding in three to four weeks, further medical evaluation is recommended. Given the location of this injury, a number of other diagnoses may be underlying.

Hamstring Tendinopathy/Tendonitis

Cause

The hamstring is vulnerable for injury at its attachment site on the ischial tuberosity, which is the bone that we sit on. The three hamstring muscles all converge to one tendon that attaches at this site. Excessive load on this tendon can cause inflammation or tendonitis. If this has been going on for a while, this tendon can thicken with scar tissue, making it harder to treat. This injury is usually due to underlying strength limitation of the posterior chain or back of the leg, especially the gluteals. This weakness causes a hamstring-dominant pattern, meaning they are not strong enough to keep up without help from the glutes. Forward hip positioning and core instability often contribute to this problem. Runners who land too far in front of their body, overextend their knees, and have increased forward hip positioning often place increased load on the hamstrings.

Presentation

Pain is felt at and just below the attachment site of the hamstring. It often feels deep and close to the sit bone. You may be able to palpate this and noticed increased pain when pushing on it. It is uncomfortable to sit and improves when standing. Running may be fine initially, but with duration symptoms increase. A shorter stride, landing closer to your body, may decrease the symptoms.

Self-Treatment

Initially the focus is on decreasing the inflammation. At the start of the injury, symptoms are normally present only when running and sitting. Limit sitting and take a brief rest from running—about five to seven days. Ice may be beneficial but due to the depth of the tissue, it may not help. Light stretching of the hamstring will help relax the tissue. An increased focus should be placed on soft-tissue mobility of the hamstring as well as massage of the tendon itself. This often needs to be done with a small ball to isolate the tendon. Long-term focus should address postural imbalance and underlying strength limitations. This often includes core stabilization along with gluteal strengthening.

In more chronic cases, eccentric strengthening has been shown through research to be beneficial. Eccentric strengthening is different from normal strengthening in that it highlights the part of the exercise where the tissue is elongating. This eccentric control is important to you as a runner because it occurs repetitively during the running gait cycle. Focusing on a reverse hamstring curl or Nordic curl works well. We will review these more in Chapter 8.

When to Seek Help

This injury is stubborn for many runners. If you have had symptoms for more than three to four weeks, you should seek further medical examination. This is essential to determine the likely biomechanical problem.

Piriformis Syndrome

Cause

Piriformis syndrome is caused by excessive tension or pressure from the piriformis muscle on the sciatic nerve beneath it. Compression of the sciatic nerve can create pain, burning, numbness, or tingling in the buttock and often radiates down the leg. It may originate from poor flexibility, but most often is rooted in biomechanical instability of the pelvis and spine. For example, an extreme pelvic tilt forward will flare the sacrum, which is where the piriformis attaches, causing increased tension. It can also be caused from external factors, such as prolonged sitting.

Presentation

Most individuals will notice deep pain in one buttock. You may also have radiating nerve sensations, or pain traveling down the back of the thigh or to any part of the lower leg or foot. Piriformis syndrome is often aggravated by prolonged sitting or driving. While running, you may notice progressive tightness in the butt, which often leads to pain and possibly to distal leg symptoms.

Self-Treatment

A short bout of rest from running may be warranted initially. This should help decrease inflammation. Second, soft-tissue mobility and flexibility can help symptoms. The focus of these should be on loosening the piriformis as well as the other hip rotators and the iliopsoas. Many find benefit in incorporating soft-tissue mobility into work or home life, such as sitting on a tennis-sized ball if sitting for longer duration. The ball should be placed at the location of the pain. If you sit or drive a lot during the day, this needs to be limited or at least broken up. Modification of posture along with frequent change in position while sitting may also help.

Long-term focus should be aimed at core stabilization. A particular target is strengthening the glutes and hip rotators. Consistency is important to translate the stability and strength to your running form.

When to Seek Help

Many people self-diagnose piriformis syndrome, but this is often inaccurate. Many refer to the pain or nerve sensations traveling down the back of the leg as sciatica, or an irritation of the sciatic nerve. Again, this is not completely accurate either. The majority of the time when these symptoms are present, they are actually stemming from the lumbar spine. Any time a nerve is affected, it is important to seek medical attention for proper diagnosis. If it is not nerve-related and only a tightness or pain that is localized to the butt, it is appropriate to treat it with flexibility and soft-tissue mobility. If symptoms begin to leave the glute region or are not improved in three to four weeks, seek further evaluation.

Snapping Hip Syndrome

Cause

Snapping hip syndrome is a term that is given to a palpable and sometimes audible snapping that occurs in the hip. Poor flexibility may be to blame for this, but it is more common in people who tend to be over-flexible. The muscle or tendon moves inside the hip as the leg swings front to back while you run. If alignment and tension are not optimal, it will slip and cause a snapping. This snapping may be asymptomatic but, with repetition or higher mileage, may become irritated.

Presentation

Snapping hip syndrome is common in younger runners, usually around high school age. It is more common in females and especially those who are flexible. These runners often have a background in dance, gymnastics, or a sport that requires a lot of flexibility.

The snap can originate from the deeper iliopsoas tendon in the front and sometimes more superficially from the TFL on the front/outer hip. It often starts as a snap that is felt occasionally, increasing to a more consistent snapping over time. Repetition of the snapping may lead to pain when the snap occurs, and then the pain lingers. It will be more noticeable walking up steps or running up hills.

Self-Treatment

Initial treatment should involve rest from running for a few days. This should decrease the snapping and inflammation. Based on the nature of this injury, flexibility of the iliopsoas, TFL, IT band, and quadriceps may be warranted. In an individual who already moves well, the focus should be on stability through the pelvis, normally to minimize an excessive forward tilt.

When to Seek Help

This injury can be quite stubborn and often, until the right rehabilitation plan is developed, slow to conquer. If focusing on the above is not yielding results in three to four weeks, further medical evaluation should be sought.

If you are in the first one to two weeks of an injury, you may benefit from a short course of an over-the-counter nonsteroidal anti-inflammatory drug, such as ibuprofen or naproxen. I am a firm believer that these are rarely the sole treatment for an injury. Anti-inflammatories may take the edge off the pain and help to decrease some of the inflammation, but the drugs treat the symptoms rather than the cause of the problem. You need to make sure you are not just masking the pain and allowing yourself to push your body into a more involved injury. If your body is in pain, there is something wrong and you need to address it.

This takes us through some of the most common running-related core injuries. It is important to recognize that this list does not include all injuries. As complex as the body is, there are other structures in the core from which symptoms could originate. If your symptoms do not align with one of these exactly, do not be alarmed. Injuries come in all shapes and sizes and often will require a medical diagnosis as well as a full-body evaluation to best direct rehabilitation of your injury. Also, many of the injuries that occur in the body may actually originate in the core, but show up elsewhere. We will explore this more in the next chapter.

Chapter 4
Other Core-Related Injuries

I hope through the first few chapters you have gained an appreciation for the complexity of your body, while remembering that we have only scratched the surface. As we start to link more areas, the chain effect that begins when the sole of the foot contacts the ground, through the leg, into the core, and through the rest of the body is quite involved. One weak link in the chain could cause a problem that shows up in another area of the body. Of the runners whom I treat every day, I estimate that at least 75 percent of their injuries, regardless of where the acute pain is, originate from their core and the mechanics that are altered by the core's limitations.

Pretend a pebble in your shoe is under the heel of your right foot. If you ran with this inside, you would land less on your heel and more on your right forefoot. This will cause your knee and hip to be more bent on this side, essentially as though your leg were shorter. This pattern places more stress on the leg and back. It may even cause an overload of the opposite leg because it is still functioning normally. Try it. Walk across the room with a normal left leg stride but on the front of the right foot. You will notice more load on the opposite limb and jarring into your back.

Now pretend the pebble is gone but you have more calf tightness on the right side than the left. This is common for those of you who drive all day and keep your right foot pointing downward on the gas.

It may not be as exaggerated as the pebble but the asymmetry causes a similar trickle up the chain when you run. The result is a back injury. The solution, though, is not treating the back. Flexibility and core work could be performed all day and although it might make it feel better, it would not fix the problem. When you returned to running, the pain would return until the calf was addressed.

In other injuries, the cause could be present in the core, but the symptoms could arise elsewhere. Take runner's knee, or patellofemoral syndrome (PFS), for example. PFS is the most common diagnosis for the runners I treat. It is a prime example of an injury that shows up one place but originates in another—often in the core. Those who have been treated for PFS say that hip strengthening was more effective than knee strengthening. That's because the problem is often mechanical and not structural.

One of the common mechanical patterns that can cause havoc for a runner originates from core inhibition. When the core is in a poor position to function, it is not powerful, rendering the glutes and hips less active. Limited activation through these areas trickles down the chain, causing a reaction: the knee falls and rotates inward, the leg has poor angulation by falling to the inside, and the foot often turns out excessively. Tracing this out to the toes, the big toe is pushed to the outside (like a bunion) and the other toes bunch up. The bottom of the foot then appears to be a calloused mess. This pattern alone could explain numerous problems. We will reference this pattern often.

In this chapter, we will cover a number of other injuries that runners face. Many of these problems originate from within the core. We will start with bone and joint injuries.

Stress Injury: Metatarsals, Tibia, Fibula

Cause

You learned about stress reactions and fractures in the previous chapter, but it is important to note that they can occur anywhere in the body. For runners, structures outside of the core are more common, such as the tibia and fibula (shin bones), or the metatarsal bones of the foot. Weakness or instability in the core can lead to poor biomechanical alignment of the lower extremities, placing excessive load on the bones.

For an example, let's focus on the metatarsals. These are the small long bones that make up the middle portion of your foot. When you push off during a running stride, they have an increased demand placed on them. A runner who has a core-inhibited pattern may put the metatarsals at a disadvantage and at risk for a stress injury.

Presentation

Stress injuries that are found in the foot and lower leg have a similar presentation to other stress injuries. In the early phases, they may be felt only later in the run or when running down hills. As they progress, symptoms may start immediately when running, eventually hindering running and causing pain with daily walking and activities. The metatarsals, tibia, and fibula are a little different than the hip in that they are more superficial. This means that often they are tender to the touch and specific in one spot. In some cases, you may even see swelling in the area.

Self-Treatment

Treatment for this is similar to a stress injury of the hip. Initial treatment is to remove the stress that has caused the injury so that it can heal. In most cases, this means rest from running and any impact activities. During this period of rest, focus on non-impact cross training as well as strengthening that does not involve stress on the involved area. In the case that underlying mechanical imbalances have caused the stress injury, appropriate core and lower extremity control exercises are important to decrease overloading of the bone.

It is critical that the underlying reason for the stress injury be identified early so that it can be treated properly.

When to Seek Help

Follow up with a medical professional quickly. Proper diagnosis will help speed recovery. Depending on the area of the stress injury, a walking boot or crutches may be needed for healing to take place. Also, the origin—be it mechanical or poor training—needs to be identified in order to rectify the true problem.

Osteoarthrosis/Osteoarthritis: Great Toe, Ankle, Knee (including Meniscus)

Cause

Osteoarthritis (OA) can be found in any joint of the body. For runners, other than the hip and spine, it is common in the great toe, ankle, or knee. Poor control through the core can lead to limitations in running mechanics and overall alignment issues of the lower body. This can lead to increased pressure on one area of the chain.

Consider the joint at the base of your big toe. This joint, known as the first MTP, can be a common area for OA to develop. A runner with a core-inhibited pattern does not align his or her foot well for the push-off phase of running. The first MTP, for the most part, is a hinge joint, meaning that it should bend in one plane—up and down in this case. If the foot is forced to turn out laterally, the big toe is pushed even more to the outside and out of proper alignment. Now the joint surfaces won't mesh well, causing increased load on one area more than another.

Stand up and point your bare feet and knees straight ahead. Bend one of your knees and lift your heel off the ground. Your big toe should bend and remain pointing in the direction of your foot and knee. Now, turn your foot out about 30 degrees, keeping your knee pointing in the straight direction (as you would when you run), and lift your heel. See how the big toe rolls more off the inside, not the pad underneath? Can you also see how it is pushed more to the outside, causing the toes to compress together? We are looking at MTP OA, but the reality is that the problem was core inhibition all along.

Degenerative change can also occur in the meniscus. There are two of these found in each knee. They are cartilaginous in nature and serve to minimize friction inside the knee and improve over-all congruency between the tibia and femur. Similar to the trickle-down effect mentioned with MTP OA, the same thing could show up in the knee. Excessive collapse inward or outward, along with excessive rotational force at the knee, can cause increased shear force and friction. This can result in fraying of the meniscus or, later on, a tear.

Presentation

OA starts with pain and swelling around a joint. It is often worse after sleeping or periods of rest. It tends to feel better when moving, within reason. After a prolonged period of time loading the joint, pain tends to increase. This pain may linger for days after the activity. In later stages, the symptoms may be more constant.

Self-Treatment

OA can't be cured, but is often able to be managed. Focus first on limiting duration and intensity of activities that are stressing the joint. Ice may be beneficial in calming down flare-ups. Long-term treatment should be directed at limiting stress on the joint through mechanical retraining.

When to Seek Help

Similar to OA of the hip and spine, if symptoms are lower level, con-tinue conservative management for up to two weeks. If symptoms increase in intensity or do not respond to conservative treatment, it is important that the pain be examined by a medical professional.

Now let's look at common soft-tissue injuries that can stem from a dysfunctional core.

Runner's Knee/Patellofemoral Syndrome

Cause

PFS is the most common injury for runners. It is normally caused by mechanical misalignment of the knee, but with strong influences from the hips, core, foot, and ankle. The patella is a floating bone found in the front of the knee. It has a small V-shaped bottom to it. This V shape articulates with a similarly grooved shape in the femur underneath. If these structures do not align well, there will be increased friction between them every time the knee bends or

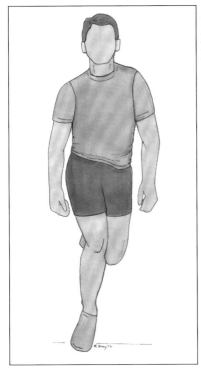

Poor lower-extremity alignment with hip drop, knee collapse inward, and lateral toe-out pattern.

The patella-femoral joint: Good alignment with base of patella aligning with groove in femur (left), and poor alignment with base of patella not aligning with groove in femur (right).

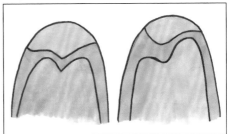

straightens. This friction over time will build to the point that the joint will heat up and inflame.

Presentation

Pain is found around the front of the knee. This most often is felt on the outer portion of the kneecap but could be anywhere around it or even deep underneath. Some may feel or hear a rubbing or grinding sensation inside the knee when they bend and straighten it. In extreme cases, the front portion of the knee may swell.

Symptoms are most often present after periods of rest, such as sitting or sleeping. After you're up and moving, the knee tends to feel better. Walking down steps or squatting will often trigger the symptoms. When running, symptoms are usually minimal early on, but increase as you go. Not running will decrease the symptoms, but it may take two to three days. Running down a hill, slowing the pace, and going up steeper up hills may also increase the pain.

If symptoms are below the kneecap and toward the inside of the top of the knee, they may be originating from a separate structure. The pes anserine is a group of tendons that funnel together on the inner portion of the knee. These tendons also have a small, fluid-filled sac known as a bursa beneath them. These structures can be inflamed by the same mechanism as PFS, creating tendonitis or bursitis.

Self-Treatment

Initially, remove the aggravating factors. This most often requires about five to seven days of rest from running. Rest along with ice calms things down but rarely fixes the problem. The key to tackling PFS long term is resolving the friction under the patella by fixing the mechanical fault.

Focus on hip strengthening and core stabilization during your rehabilitation program. Flexibility, along with soft-tissue mobility of the quadriceps, TFL/IT band, and hip flexors, may also be beneficial.

As these areas improve, it is important that strengthening is tied into retraining the alignment of the knee. This may involve proprioception, or balance retraining, along with retraining the lower extremity alignment during squats or lunges.

All of this will also be indicated in the treatment of pes anserine dysfunctions. In addition, soft-tissue mobility of the inner thigh and quad should also be performed regularly.

It is also important to recognize that a biomechanical problem with your running stride could also be the primary factor. Initial retraining should focus on landing more lightly and often with more bend in the knee. This often reforms you from a heel striker to landing in a mid-foot position closer to the body.

When to Seek Help

As stubborn and reoccurring as PFS can be, it is essential that the underlying cause be identified early. If you have followed the above and are not seeing improvement in three to four weeks, seek further medical evaluation. I strongly recommend a gait and running assessment for anyone who has followed a more conventional pathway without results. I see way too many runners who have been doing strength and flexibility exercises for months—or even years—who have not had improvement. Often, subtle gait mechanics can lead to ongoing PFS.

In the older population or in more extreme cases, OA may be underlying and therefore causing increased friction in the knee. If you notice rubbing, grinding, or swelling in the knee, OA may have an influence on PFS. This should be examined by a health professional.

Iliotibial Band Syndrome (ITBS)

Cause

Most runners have heard of iliotibial or IT band syndrome. This is another common diagnosis. It occurs from excessive stress or friction over the IT band and the underlying bony prominence on the outside of the knee. This can be caused by poor lower extremity biomechanical alignment, similar to PFS and/or poor running biomechanics. If the knee rotates and collapses inward during running, an increased load is placed on the outer portion of the knee. This load increases the amount of friction in the IT band as it slides over the bone. With higher friction and more repetition comes an increased risk of inflammation. Runners who extend their knee more fully when landing will also cause excessive load on the IT band.

Presentation

Pain is present and often able to be palpated over the outer portion of the knee. It is normally close to the bony prominence that is felt most laterally at the height of the patella. Pain is normally not present at rest but may increase when beginning to move after sitting or sleeping. Some individuals may have lower-level symptoms when sitting cross-legged. Similar to PFS, symptoms normally feel better after you are moving. Pain tends to build the more you run. If this has been going on for a while, the pain will often force you to stop. Going downhill or more slowly tends to increase symptoms. Running up hills or at faster intervals will often feel a little better.

Self-Treatment

If symptoms are lower level, initial treatment can focus on soft-tissue mobility of the IT band and surrounding soft tissues. This, in conjunction with ice, may lessen symptoms to a level such that you are able to continue running. If symptoms are higher level or have been going on for a while, a period of rest may be necessary. Start with five to seven days, along with the above treatment to decrease the inflammation and pain. In addition to soft-tissue mobility of the IT band, hip flexor, and TFL, flexibility is important. Later treatment should include hip strength and core stabilization. Again, it is important to have a running gait assessment. Many runners extend their knee too much when they run, placing more friction on the IT band than needed. Patients who minimize the overextension in their knee while running often resolve symptoms completely.

When to Seek Help

If symptoms have been present for three to four weeks or more, you should seek profession medical attention. This will confirm the diagnosis and guide your treatment in the right direction.

Patella Tendinopathy/Tendonitis

Cause

The patella tendon is just below the kneecap. This is the tendon that attaches the quadriceps muscle group via the patella to the tibia. It is felt as a thick band that runs vertically. The quadriceps work closely in conjunction with the gluteals to help absorb impact when contacting the ground during running. If strength is not adequate to control this force, often the patella tendon will become overloaded and inflamed. If this pattern continues for a longer period of time, the tendon will often thicken with scar tissue, making rehabilitation harder. If you have poor lower-body control and alignment during running and loading-based exercises, you're placing more demand on the tendon.

Presentation

Pain and, in more extreme cases, swelling is present around the front of the knee, just below the kneecap. The patella tendon is most often tender when palpating it. Symptoms are often present when bending the knee while squatting, kneeling, or trying to stretch your quadriceps. Pain normally increases when running, and minimal difference is felt between the terrain and pace that you are running.

Self-Treatment

Initial treatment should consist of light flexibility work to the quadriceps and hip flexors. Soft-tissue mobility to these areas and self-massage to the tendon will also help. Perform massage up and down, as well as back and forth on the tendon. It may be a little sore when you do this, but it should feel better afterward. If symptoms are increasing while running and have been going on for a while, it is important to rest for a short duration. During this time, ice will be important to help calm inflammation.

With most of these cases, the patella tendon has been aggravated for a while before a runner begins to treat it. As a result, a long-term plan should focus on hip strength, especially of the gluteals. Also, an eccentric quadriceps strengthening program has been shown to help more chronic cases. This is a similar approach to the treatment of the proximal hamstring tendon, although a different exercise. It can be set up using a single leg-lowering squat to a chair or higher surface. Perform the lowering phase only. When rising from the seated position, help yourself with your hands and other leg.

When to Seek Help

If you have focused on the above or symptoms have been going on for three to four weeks, seek further medical evaluation. Based on the level of inflammation, a longer duration of rest may be indicated. Also, more extensive strengthening and stabilization work may need to be included in the treatment plan.

Achilles Tendinopathy/Tendonitis

Cause

The Achilles tendon attaches the muscles that make up the calf complex to the back of the heel. This seems pretty far down the leg from the core. However, this tendon has a close link to what is happening higher up the chain in the core. Think of pushing off the ground to do a jump with your knees straight and then bent. If your knees are locked, you are not going to be able to jump very high because all of the power has to come from the calf. If you bend the knees, however, you are able to recruit some of the larger muscles up the chain such as your quadriceps and glutes. A runner who is not recruiting his glutes well drives more from his calf. This ultimately will overload the Achilles and increase risk for injury.

Poor lower-extremity alignment can also increase load on the Achilles. Think of someone who rolls her foot too far to the inside. This over-pronation causes a bowing of the Achilles, which does not allow an efficient push-off, and thus overloading.

Presentation

Pain is present lengthwise in the Achilles, but most often localized to the base just above the heel. Along with pain, the tendon often feels tight. These symptoms are amplified first thing in the morning when getting out of bed, or after periods of inactivity. Normally, the symptoms will decrease with movement. When running, the symptoms tend to get worse with duration and higher-intensity running.

Self-Treatment

Initial treatment should focus on soft-tissue mobility and light calf flexibility exercises. Along with this, ice may be beneficial to decrease acute symptoms. Depending on the severity of the inflammation, rest may be necessary.

Similar to more chronic injuries of the hamstring and patella tendon, eccentric strengthening can help as well. This can be performed by using a calf raise off a small block of wood or step. Remember, with eccentric exercises, the tissue is worked only in the lowering movement. In this case, a calf raise would be performed with both feet along with upper body assistance by pushing off a table or other firm object. The involved leg would then perform a slow reverse calf raise, meaning the lowering motion. Then you would again use the other foot and hands to help return to the high starting position.

When to Seek Help

If symptoms are not improving with the above after three to four weeks, it is important that you seek further medical examination. Based on the level of involvement, alternative treatment may be indicated before returning to running. Also, as in most of these injuries, a gait and running assessment is likely needed.

Shin Splints/Medial Tibial Stress Syndrome

Cause

Shin splints are extremely common among the middle and high school-aged running population. They are caused most often by excessive stress to the muscle that attaches to the tibia. This could be from poor biomechanics, such as hard and excessive heel striking, overuse, or underlying strength limitations. Many younger athletes have bodies that are still developing. Often, they are growing fast and their strength is not keeping up with their height. When they run, limitations in strength and mechanics stress the muscle attaching to the tibia. This excessive stress causes irritation at the attachment to the bone.

Presentation

Most shin splints are felt in the lower portion of the inner shin. This is often quite tender to touch. Depending on the severity, pain may be present early in a run or may come on more gradually. In more severe cases, pain is present when walking and usually increases when walking down steps.

Self-Treatment

Rest for five to seven days along with ice should help to calm down the symptoms initially. In some cases, an off-the-shelf shoe insert may help minimize stress on the shin. A long-term plan needs to focus on reeducating running mechanics to limit stress on the tibia. This often includes retraining a shorter stride length and minimizing an aggressive heel-strike pattern. It is also essential that core stabilization and hip strength be maximized. This will help to improve control, aiding in better running mechanics and less stress on the shin.

When to Seek Help

If the shin splints have been increasing in intensity or are becoming more specific to one spot in the shin, seek further medical examination. If left untreated, shin splints could develop into stress injuries of the tibia.

Posterior Tibialis Tendinopathy/Tendonitis and Peroneal Tendinopathy/Tendonitis

Cause

I'm grouping the above together because their relationship to the core is often similar in nature.

The posterior tibialis muscle is found deep in the lower leg. It turns into a tendon that crosses behind the inner ankle bone and wraps underneath the foot. Its primary function is to control the amount the foot pronates or rolls to the inside. Limited core control and strength can cause excessive pronation of the foot, stressing this tendon and leading to tendonitis.

Similarly, the peroneals are a group of three muscles found in the outer leg. They have tendons crossing behind and in front of the outer ankle bone. They aid in controlling the amount the foot rolls outward. In the case of a higher-arched or supinated foot, these tendons are stressed more, which may lead to an inflammation of these tendons.

Presentation

With posterior tibialis tendonitis, pain is most often found and palpable across the inner ankle and possibly bottom of the foot. Peroneal tendonitis typically presents with pain across the outer ankle wrapping down to the outer foot. Both injuries tend to be aggravated more with duration of running and often with uneven ground. With more exacerbated cases, symptoms may be present with walking or standing as well.

Self-Treatment

Rest and ice initially should help to calm down the acute inflammation. An off-the-shelf shoe insert may also help to provide some short-term relief. If symptoms are lower level and running is impacted minimally, try to stay on surfaces that keep your foot level left to right, such as a track or back road. Higher crowned roads or uneven trails will often aggravate these problems. Soft-tissue mobility to the affected tissue, inner or outer leg, will help to relieve symptoms. Long-term, focus on controlling the excessive movement of the foot in either direction. This is done through a series of flexibility and strength exercises, and most often running mechanics retraining.

When to Seek Help

As with many of the other soft-tissue injuries, if your symptoms are not responding to the above or are increasing, seek medical attention in three to four weeks. Inflammation that has been lingering for a while can cause scar tissue within the tendon that may need to be addressed with alternative treatment. In more severe and longer-lasting cases, tearing may occur in these tendons.

Plantar Fasciosis/Fasciitis

Cause

The final injury that we will look at is plantar fasciosis. I call this fasciosis because I rarely see a true case of plantar fasciitis in my medical practice. Most patients do not seek medical attention for this until the symptoms have been lasting for weeks or months. Often by this point, it is not just irritated at lower levels but often quite painful and chronic.

The plantar fascia is a band of tissue that extends from the heel bone to the front of the foot. It helps to maintain arch control and stiffen the foot for improved push-off power when running. Poor hip strength or position can cause over-pronation or a lateral toe-out pattern during running. This places excessive load on the plantar fascia and minimizes the ability of the foot to push off in an efficient manner. This initially leads to inflammation in the plantar fascia and escalates to small micro-tears and degenerative change of the fascia.

Presentation

Plantar fascia injuries tend to follow a classic presentation with pain in the origin of the fascia on the bottom of the heel bone. Often this pain is present on the inside of the bottom of the heel. Pain tends to be absent when off your feet, but increases upon rising, especially first thing in the morning. Normally, the pain will improve in a matter of minutes after walking. When running, the pain may or may not be present. In cases where pain does come on, it usually increases with duration. If pain is not present during, often it will be more noticeable afterward with the transition out of sedentary positions.

Self-Treatment

This can be a stubborn injury for runners but if treated appropriately, it can be fixed. If you are experiencing plantar fascia pain for the first time, I would tackle it with the basics. Perform light stretching and soft-tissue mobility of the plantar fascia and calf. Regular icing and a short stint of activity modification should also help in controlling the symptoms. If symptoms have been going on for multiple weeks or this is an exacerbation of an old injury, the basics may not be enough. Hip flexor stretching, glute strengthening, and core stabilization may be essential in controlling the foot better. By improving these and working toward controlling foot alignment with walking and running, symptoms should diminish over time. Also, reoccurrence should be minimized if the true underlying cause is identified.

When to Seek Help

I am a strong advocate for having this evaluated early. It's common for runners to wait too long for treatment, which makes it a stubborn and frustrating fix. If you are someone who has experienced this in the past and it starts to rear its head again, seek medical help. If these symptoms are presenting for the first time, follow the above for one to two weeks, but if symptoms are worsening, have a medical professional determine an appropriate treatment regime before it evolves into something more chronic.

It is important to recognize that flexibility, soft-tissue mobility, strength, stability, and mechanics are essential to the rehabilitation of an injury. However, overuse or overtraining can also be culprits. Runners are highly motivated individuals who like to push themselves. Take the most perfectly fit, well-conditioned, and biomechanically sound runner. If this individual increases mileage too fast or pushes too hard with training, she may become injured. In a case like this, exercises for flexibility and strengthening may help to minimize symptoms, but until proper rest and modification of the running progression are implemented, she will continue to have problems.

We have now covered the majority of the most common running-related injuries. The information provided should serve as a reference to help direct care. It is not a substitute for a thorough medical examination. If your symptoms are not improving or are accompanied by symptoms elsewhere in the body, follow up with your primary care physician to discuss an appropriate plan for treatment.

The self-treatment that is listed in these chapters provides a starting point to tackle these injuries. The better you understand yourself, the more you will be able to guide your own treatment. Even more importantly, the more you know about your body, the more you will be able to prevent injury. Let's take some time to assess your current level of flexibility, core stability, and movement patterns.

Chapter 5

Runner's Core Assessment

Most runners who feel an onset of pain, think about injuries, or even just have a general goal of strengthening their core turn to the Internet or a magazine for answers. These sources are loaded with training plans and exercises that are easy to implement. The problem is that these plans are not specific to you.

Think about two scenarios. First, look at a high school girl who is a gymnast and ballet dancer and decides she wants train for a 5K. Online she finds a basic program for her core. It involves hip stretching and strengthening. She starts training. Does this individual, who is already doing gymnastics, really need to do more flexibility exercises? Does she even need the strengthening? These exercises may be a waste of her time. In reality, she may need to simply learn better running posture, which she will not achieve through her new program.

Second, consider a forty-year-old man, who travels weekly for his job and otherwise finds himself desk-bound in the office, and who decides to train for a 5K. He looks online for a conditioning program for his core and comes up with hip strengthening and core stabilization. After a number of weeks he feels that the exercises are working, because they are getting easier to do. But an individual who is sitting all day and traveling most weeks is likely lacking mobility. He may need to include some movement and flexibility.

In order to determine the areas that you need to focus on, you need to assess your core. That's what this chapter is about. As part of the core assessment, we will look at multiple areas: core stability, general strength, flexibility, mobility, balance, breath control, and dynamic control. These are all essential building blocks to complete a well-rounded core. You may look at a few of these tests and think that they don't relate to the core, but remember that your core is a complex chain and only as strong as the weakest link.

The most important component of a runner's core examination is a gait assessment. It is still too easy for runners to work for months on stretching and strengthening when this may not be the problem at all. It may be the way they are running. One of the reasons that gait assessment is not looked at more is because it is more costly and requires an expert.

To perform an assessment on your own, you will need a stopwatch, an assistant (or mirror) for feedback, and a video camera. Also, this assessment should be performed barefoot.

Remember as you go through these tests that quality is more important than quantity. Muscling through a test to get a higher score may seem like a good idea, but it really only skews the results that are designed to help. This assessment will take about thirty minutes, but will save you hours in the long run. Keep track of your score along the way. It is also important to note why you scored yourself the way you did to focus on the quality in the exercises. Each test will be scored as zero, one, or two. Do not perform a test if you have pain trying it; instead, score it as a zero. Take off your shoes and let's get going.

Part A: Breath Control

Test 1—Breathing

Purpose

This test will assess your pattern of breathing and your ability to control it. This is an essential foundation for optimal positioning of the core during exercises and running.

Set Up

Lie with your back flat on the ground with your knees bent and your feet flat on the ground. Place both hands on your mid-chest so that your thumbs are on your lower ribs, palms are on the sides, and fingers over your abdomen. Take five relaxed breaths in and out. Feel for rise and fall of the ribs in comparison to the abdomen.

Scoring

  0: Ribs are flared up to the ceiling and are predominant movers during breathing.
  1: Ribs are fairly level and move along with abdomen equally during breathing.
  2: Ribs are fairly level and move minimally with abdomen moving more during breathing.

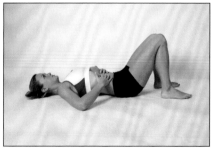

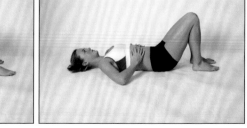

Test 1, Breathing Score 0.   **Test 1, Breathing Score 2.**

Part B: Movement—Flexibility/Mobility

Test 2—Squat

Purpose

The squat test will assess your ankle, hip, and spine mobility. It is also a general reflection of your overall movement patterns, which is crucial for core control and running biomechanics.

Set Up

Stand with your feet shoulder-width apart and pointing straight ahead. Place both arms straight in front of you so that they are parallel to the floor. Squat down like you are sitting into a chair, as low as you can go. Make sure your heels stay on the ground. Pay attention to how low you can go, the alignment of your back, and which direction your feet and knees point.

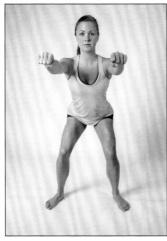

Test 2, Squat Score 0.

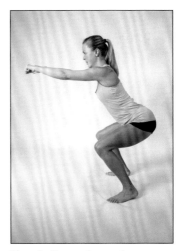

Test 2, Squat Score 1.

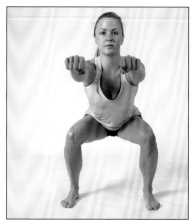

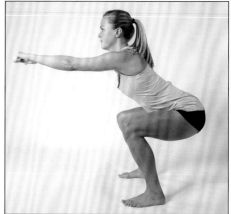

Test 2, Squat Score 2 (front view).   **Test 2, Squat Score 2 (side view).**

Scoring

  0: Your hips do not drop below your knees.
  1: Your hips drop close to the height of your knees, but your heels elevate off the ground, your feet and/or knees deviate from pointing straight ahead.
  2: Your hips drop below your knees while your feet and knees point forward.

Test 3—Half Kneeling

Purpose

The half-kneeling test will assess the mobility of your pelvis to get into a running position, with one leg in front and one leg behind. It will also look at your big toe and ankle mobility, which are additional key components for a better-aligned runner.

Set Up

You will need a wall. Place one knee on the ground and the other knee bent in front of you with the foot flat on the ground and facing the wall. Your big toe should be close to the wall. The foot in the back should be vertical with your toes tucked underneath. Perform a light tuck of your pelvis so that your spine is not overly arched, and hold. Shift your hips and knee forward, maintaining a vertical posture. If your knee comfortably touches the wall without your heel lifting up, move your foot away from the wall a little more. Find the point where your knee can touch the wall but just before your front foot heel elevates or turns outward, or you lose your hip position. Make note of the distance from your big toe to the wall. The goal of this test is to see how far you can get your toes from the wall with good alignment. Also take note of how close to horizontal the back foot's great toe is. The number of degrees does not need to be measured—a rough visual will do. Then perform the same test with the other leg forward.

Scoring

**Both sides must meet all criteria in a category to receive that score; if not, score with the lower number.

0: You have less than half a fist width from your great toe to the wall. Tightness in your hips limits your ability to perform this test. Your back toe is between vertical and 30 degrees from vertical (0–30 degrees).

1: You have between half a fist width and a full fist width from your great toe to the wall. You have minimal to no tightness in your hips during the test. Your back toe is 30–70 degrees.

2: You have a fist width or more from your big toe to the wall. You have no tightness in your hips during the test. Your back toe is flexed to 70 degrees or more.

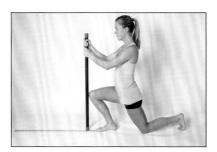

Test 3, Half Kneeling set-up. Ruler showing distance from big toe to base of the bar/wall.

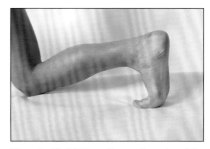

Test 3, Half Kneeling, showing big toe angle of 80 degrees, score of 2.

Part C: Core Stabilization

Test 4—Trunk Flexor Endurance

Purpose

This test will assess core stability, focusing on the front of the core and its endurance. This test is quality-driven and is a reflection of how well you can maintain appropriate hip and spine postural control necessary for running.

Set Up

Lie with your back flat on the ground. Place both hands slightly under the small of your back. Press your back into your hands and hold this position. Raise your head and shoulders slightly off the ground. Now raise your legs in the air so that your hips and knees are both bent to 90 degrees. Time how long you can hold this position, paying close attention to maintaining your back against your hands. Stop the test if your legs, head, or shoulders drop, or if your lower back begins to arch up.

Scoring

0: A time of 0–44 seconds
1: A time of 45–89 seconds
2: A time of 90 seconds or
     more

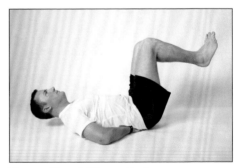

Test 4, Trunk Flexor Endurance set-up.

Test 5—Side Plank (Left and Right)

Purpose

This test will assess core stability, focusing on the sides of the core and their endurance. These areas are key to maintaining lower extremity and trunk control during the stance phase of your gait.

Set Up

Lie on your side with your top leg slightly in front of your bottom leg. Place the forearm on the down side against the ground and under your shoulder. Raise your hips off the ground, balancing on your feet and arm. Maintain a straight line along your feet, hips, spine, and head. Be careful not to let your hips sag toward the ground. Time how long you can hold this position, stopping if your hips drop or lift up, or if your body starts to move forward or back. Then repeat on your other side.

Scoring

**Both sides must be within the time frame. If they are not, score yourself with the lower time.

0: A time of 0-29 seconds

1: A time of 30-59 seconds

2: A time of 60 seconds or more

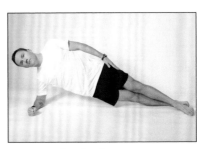

Test 5, Side Plank set-up.

Test 6—Plank

Purpose

This test will assess global core stability and endurance, including all aspects of the hips and core. It serves as a good baseline to track overall core endurance.

Set Up

Lie on the ground flat on your stomach. Place your forearms flat on the ground with your elbows under your shoulders. Lift your body off of the ground and make a straight line through your ankles, knees, hips, shoulders, and head.

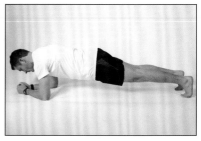

Test 6, Plank set-up.

Focus on keeping your stomach and glutes tight, trying to minimize the amount your stomach sags toward the ground. Time how long you can hold this position, stopping if your hips drop or lift up. Also stop if your stomach sags.

Scoring

  0: A time of 0–44 seconds
  1: A time of 45–89 seconds
  2: A time of 90 seconds or more

Test 7—Shoulder Touch Push-Up

Purpose

This test will assess rotational core stability. Rotational stabilization is essential to a runner, given the counter-movement that occurs in the hips and torso during each running stride.

Set Up

Start in a push-up position with your hands on the ground at shoulder width and your feet shoulder width apart. Keep your body straight. Slowly take one hand and touch the opposite shoulder. Then perform this on the other side. Repeat a total of five repetitions for each shoulder. If you are unable to perform this, widen your foot width to three feet apart and try again. This test should

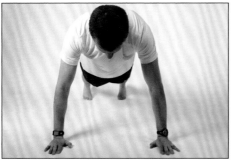 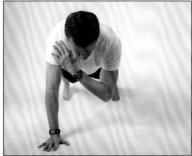

Test 7, Shoulder Touch Push-Up set-up, start point.   Test 7, Shoulder Touch Push-Up set-up, end point.

be performed slowly, maintaining torso and shoulders level to the ground during.

Scoring

  0: Unable to maintain body position and perform five slow touches to each side with wide foot stance.
  1: Able to perform five slow touches with wide foot stance but unable to perform five touches with narrow foot stance.
  2: Able to perform five slow touches or more with feet at shoulder width.

Part D: General Strength

Test 8—Single Leg Calf Raise

Purpose

This test assesses isolated calf strength. Calf strength is essential to dampening impact during the initial contact and loading response phases of your gait and is also important with push-off during terminal stance. Limitations or imbalances here can cause overload or increased torque of the core.

Set Up

Stand vertically, holding on to a stable object with one hand to help your balance. Take one foot off of the ground. Raise up on your forefoot on the other side, lifting your heel off the ground, as high as you are able to. Then lower your heel back to the ground until it lightly touches. Repeat this up/down motion at a slow and controlled pace without taking breaks. Count the number you can perform on each side. Stop the test if you need to rest.

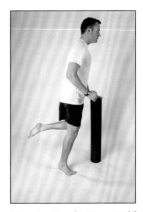

Test 8, Single-Leg Calf Raise set-up.

Scoring

**Both sides must achieve the same level of scoring; otherwise, score yourself with the lower score.

   0: Repetitions between 0–9
   1: Repetitions between 10–24
   2: Repetitions more than 25

Test 9—Single-Leg Squat

Purpose

This test will assess your overall isolated single-leg strength. It also will assess your core's ability to control your single-limb strength during movement. This is one of the best tests for a runner because running is a single-leg activity—both legs are never on the ground at one time. It is necessary for each leg to be able to accept the stress from body weight and the impact on the ground. It is even more important that the core can appropriately control the alignment of the leg on the ground.

Set Up

First, calculate one-third of your height. You will be using this height for the depth of your single-leg squat.

Height (inches) _____ x .33 = _____ Height of Object (inches)

Next, find an object at this height, such as a low coffee table or chair, placing the necessary number of books or other small objects on top of this until it achieves the calculated height. Now, line yourself up in front of this so that when you squat down, your hips will reach backward and are able to lightly touch the top object. Now that you have the set-up complete, start the test.

Start with one leg. With your foot facing straight ahead, perform as many controlled squats as you can. Make sure that your knee points forward and your hips are level and squared off in the direction that you are facing. One full rep will be counted if you lightly touch your butt to the measured object and then fully stand back up with your knee straight. If you lose your balance and need to use your foot or hand for assistance, the repetition is not counted. A

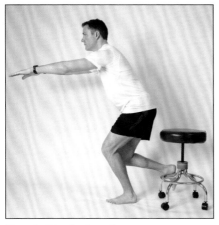

Test 9, Single-Leg Squat set-up.

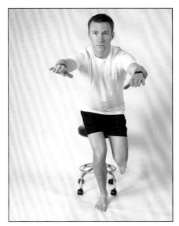

Test 9, Single-Leg Squat showing good alignment of foot and knee for a score of 1 or 2.

mirror or short video of you performing this may be helpful to see your lower-body alignment.

Scoring

0: Total repetitions 0-9 and challenged to control proper foot and knee alignment.

1: Total repetitions 10-19 with good alignment of foot and knee.

2: Total repetitions 20 or more with good alignment of foot and knee.

Part E: Control—Static and Dynamic

Test 10—Single-Leg Balance

Purpose

This will assess your static running balance. Balance is a reflection of how well your body works and how fast it is able to react. The core is essential in stabilization to minimize extraneous movement and improve control. The carryover to running is direct because every stride involves a brief period of balance on one leg while it goes through the stance phase.

Set Up

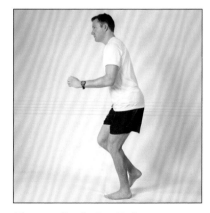

Stand on one leg with your knee bent to approximately 30 degrees. Hold your arms in a position like you are running. Slightly shift your weight forward to the front portion of the foot but keep your heel on the ground. Time how long you are able to hold this position, stopping if you lose balance more than

Test 10, Single-Leg Balance set-up.

a little or have to put your other foot down. Then repeat this test on the other side.

Scoring

**Both sides must be within the time frame. If they are not, score yourself with the lower time.

   0: A time of 0–44 seconds

   1: A time of 45–89 seconds

   2: A time of 90 seconds or more

Test 11—Single-Leg Triple Hop

Purpose

This test will assess symmetry of single-leg dynamic control. Symmetry is essential for overall balance and stability throughout the body during running. Dynamic control on one leg is important to be able to load the leg when running in the most efficient and least injury-prone way.

Set Up

Find an area where you have some space in front of you. Mark a spot on the ground as a starting point and put your toes there. Pick one leg and perform three single-leg hops forward as far as you can, sticking the landing for a second between each hop. Mark where your toes land and measure that distance. Make sure that you are in control. If you put your other foot down for balance, you need

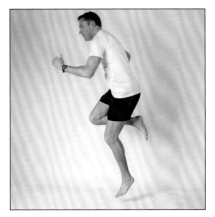

Test 11, Single-Leg Triple Hop showing technique during one hop.

to retest. Perform three trials on each side and record the farthest series of three jumps on each side.

If able, have someone watch or film you from the front or rear. Observe which way your foot points, the direction your knee moves, and how level your hips are when you push off and contact the ground.

Scoring

Divide the length of the shorter distance in feet by the length of the longer distance in feet to get A (shorter distance/longer distance = A).

Multiply A by 100 to get B (A x 100 = B).

Subtract B from 100 to get C, the percent difference between sides (100 - B = C).

0: C is 20% or more
1: C is 10–19%
2: C is 0–9%

Part F—Running Mechanics

Test 12—Running Mechanics Self-Screen

Purpose

The above tests have assessed various areas of core stability, core strength, and core control. We now must put these into action, because a runner's core self-assessment would not be complete without looking at the run itself.

Have you watched yourself run before? If not, this is extremely important. We are not all experts in gait analysis but you won't need to be for this test. I am amazed when I film patients running in the clinic and show them the results. I hear all too often, "Is that what I really look like when I run? Do my arms do that? I thought I was landing on my toes, not my heels." Most of these findings are quite evident to anyone watching and require only a short video and a little bit of your time.

Set Up

Put your running footwear on for this test. A treadmill or open area with about thirty feet is needed. If you are on a treadmill, have your assistant take a ten-second video of you from the front, side, and back. If you are doing this outside, have your helper film a thirty-foot distance of the same angles.

Now, watch these videos looking for red flags:

- Do your hands swing past your midline or belly button?
- Are your feet pointing anywhere other than straight ahead?
- Do your knees aim in a direction other than forward?
- Are your hips not level or your belt line not parallel to the ground?
- Does your trunk rotate excessively from side to side?
- Are you bent forward at the waist?
- Does your foot contact the ground far in front of your body?
- Do you land hard on your heels with your toes elevated in the air?
- Do you bounce up and down a lot?

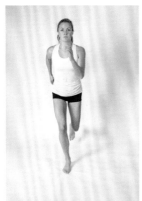 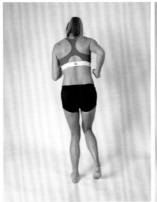 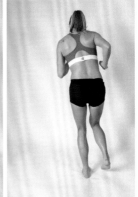

Good alignment of trunk, hips, knees, and feet.

Poor knee control with collapse across the body.

Poor trunk control with excessive movement laterally.

Scoring

This is a qualitative test and will not be scored. The red flags that are listed above serve as a starting point for the assessment. If you notice any of these, do they seem subtle or grossly out of place? Degree is important. Also, do you notice any asymmetries between right and left? Running should be symmetric, and differences between sides may reflect an underlying limitation and a precursor for injury.

This is not designed to take the place of a professional video gait assessment by any means. It is an exercise that is aimed at allowing a runner to watch herself. You will learn a lot in thirty seconds of video, which should heighten your awareness during running. If you are looking for a more in-depth analysis and feedback, I strongly recommend following up with a specialist in running gait assessments.

Final Scoring

Test #	Value (Right / Left)		Test Score (0,1,2)
1: Breath Control			
2: Squat			
3: Half Kneeling	R	L	
4: Trunk Flexor Endurance			
5: Side Plank	R	L	
6: Plank			
7: Shoulder Touch Push-Up			
8: Single-Leg Calf Raise	R	L	
9: Single-Leg Squat	R	L	
10: Single-Leg Balance	R	L	
11: Single-Leg Triple Hop	R	L	
	TOTAL SCORE		

For tests with Right and Left values, select the lower number if the two values are different.

Total Score Interpretation

0—10: Poor—Good thing you did this test. By developing a plan to address your limitations you will see improvements in your core and benefit to your running.

11—13: Below Average—You have a few areas to improve to get back in the middle of the pack. With a focused plan you will start to advance one step at a time.

14—16: Average—You are right in the middle of the pack. With a little focus on some of your limitations, you can take one more step toward the leaders.

17—19: Good—You will need to improve a couple of areas, but otherwise are doing well.

20—22: Excellent—Nice work! Fine-tune the areas of weakness and keep up your maintenance.

As you analyze the results of each of the tests, it is important to not only look at the final number, but also the quality of movement in each test. Quality is just as important as quantity, but much harder to assess. Also, take special note of the symmetry between the two sided tests: half kneel, side plank, single-leg calf raise, single-leg squat, single-leg balance, and single-leg hop. These numbers should be the same or close to each other. If they vary greatly, focus on balancing these during your training.

These results will help you to devise a plan to maximize your overall core health. The results are also an excellent reference point to track progress. Hold on to these and come back and reassess in a few months. You will see steady improvement. Reevaluate at the start of each running season or new training plan. This helps to identify limitations or imbalances before they are problematic.

In the next chapter, we will use your results to build a healthier core.

Chapter 6

Core Positioning and Breathing

What did you think about Test One on breathing in Chapter 5? Was this test awkward to perform? Did you wonder why breathing is the first test in a core book? Most people think of a sit-up or a plank as the best tests to assess their core, but it is much deeper than this. Your core's position, body's posture, and the way you breathe have a direct influence on your ability to activate and stabilize through your core when you are running.

Start with respiration or breathing—this is your lifeline. Breathing is how you get oxygen, vital to living, into the cells of your body and also expel carbon dioxide, which is harmful to you. Oxygen is essential for cell function. It is used in the production of energy in order for your body to do work. When a higher demand is placed on the body, such as running, more oxygen is required. So to do this, you need to increase the rate at which you are breathing and also maximize the volume of air exchange on each breath.

Think about the last time you were running and began to fatigue. Your breathing became more labored. This is natural. As your fitness improves, the point at which you fatigue is delayed until later in your run or at faster paces. But what if you could do more to delay fatigue? Because breathing is directly tied to fatigue, let's focus on this.

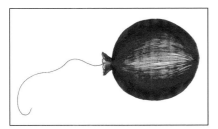

Balloon representation of lungs when expanded.

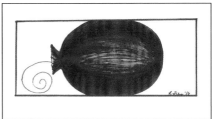

Balloon constrained by box, similar to rib cage in the body.

Every time you take a breath, an amount of oxygen fills your lungs in preparation for air exchange. If your lungs are able to expand and acquire more air, they will provide more oxygen to the body, hence more energy. Your lungs are like balloons. The air goes in, the balloon expands. Now, what if the balloon were placed inside a small box? You would still be able to put air in, but when the balloon reached the size of the box, it would be constrained and unable to expand more. That box is your rib cage. It has some elasticity to it, but it can stretch only so far, which means you need other avenues to fill your lungs.

So, we turn to the diaphragm. This is the large, flat muscle just below the lungs and is the top of the core, or the box. Its role is to draw the air into the lungs. The diaphragm looks like a parachute in its resting position. When it contracts, it flattens downward. This action decreases the pressure and increases the amount of space in the thoracic cavity where the lungs are found, triggering them to fill with air. The more the diaphragm is able to flatten, the deeper the breath will be. Position of your core is key.

Recall the open scissors position from Chapter 2, in which your pelvis is tipped forward and your lower rib cage is elevated upward. In the open scissors posture, the diaphragm is still a dome, but rather than facing downward it is more forward. In contrast, the pelvic floor musculature also faces more forward instead of remaining flat. If the diaphragm and pelvic floor contract in this position, all of the pressure will be pushed forward. If you squeeze a jelly donut with both hands, and your hands are angled as you press them together, the jelly will squeeze toward the open side of your hands. But if you make your hands parallel, then pressure is applied in all directions and the jelly could ooze out everywhere. The diaphragm and pelvic floor act similarly and should be relatively parallel and able to oppose one another for enhanced core stability.

Neutral Core

I must mention "neutral core" here. This is the position where your core is well-aligned with the pelvis, level left to right, minimally tipped forward, the lumbar and thoracic spine have small, natural curves, and thus the rib cage is level on the bottom. Internalize this neutral core position because it will be important not only while you run but with almost all of the exercises that you will be performing to improve your core. Without this position, you will not maximize your conditioning.

To help achieve a neutral core, use this simple reset exercise.

Lie on your back with your hips and knees flexed to 90 degrees. Place your feet on a chair or a wall to support them. Feel just under your lower back to assess the amount of space between your back and the floor. You want this to be minimal. Also, feel your lower rib cage in this position. Is it fairly level with the rest of your ribs or is it protruding upward? You want it to be fairly level. Start by performing a small tuck of the pelvis. Think of lifting your sacrum while you lift up on the front of the hips. Your lower back should flatten as you do this. Now, depress your lower ribs slightly down. You should now be in a neutral position. If

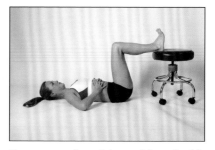

Core neutral position achieved with hips and knees flexed to 90 degrees.

this is easy, perform this exercise with your legs flat on the ground and then progress to standing.

Now that you understand the neutral core position, we will focus on breathing. True core stability starts with air. In Chapter 1, you read about the core musculature and how it is not complete without the air inside. The pressure inside the core is what allows you to stabilize. If one muscle of the core contracts in isolation, it creates movement instead of stability. If all the muscles contract together, a stability cascade begins, but they need to contract against something. In this case it is air. Think of a soft, air-filled ball. If you poked it with one finger it would feel spongy and your finger would sink in. But if you pressed your hands on either side, the ball would increase in pressure and become firmer. You'd feel more resistance if you pressed your finger into it. It's the same with your core.

When you breathe in, your diaphragm contracts to fill the lungs with air. With your core in the right position, your abdomen will increase in pressure. This is known as intra-abdominal pressure, or IAP. You want to maximize IAP to improve overall core stability. To do this, you must start in the correct position, breathe efficiently, and then balance the contraction among your diaphragm, pelvis, and trunk musculature. If this is all done fluidly, then IAP will be greater and you will achieve more stability from your core.

Infants do a great job of this. Next time you are around a baby, watch her breathing. You will notice that babies have a little belly that tends to be the primary mover as they breathe. The majority of their breath is coming from an efficient movement of the lungs and diaphragm. This increases pressure and stability in their core. If the breath does not create the pressure exchange well, you end up with a more apical breathing pattern. Apical breathing occurs when the upper chest is dominant with movement as you breathe. In a relaxed state, you should not see this breathing pattern.

Next time you are out for a run with friends, watch the way they breathe. You will notice that more often than not, someone who is floating along effortlessly will have a relaxed breathing pattern. There will be minimal movement in his upper chest, shoulders, and back. This is how it should be for day-to-day activity and relaxed exercise. In contrast, look at the person who is struggling as he runs. You will notice this person trying hard to get more air and see expansion higher in his chest. This is not efficient. The person is likely pushing his limits and is going to need to rest shortly because an apical breathing pattern is hard to sustain.

I like to think of this as the fight-or-flight breathing. If you were out for a run and a bear began to chase you, I expect that you are going to start to suck air into your body any way you can. It is similar to hyperventilation and is not sustainable. Therefore, you need to perform diaphragmatic breathing well while you are running for overall efficiency and improved performance.

Diaphragmatic Breathing

Start in the same position as the previous exercise, with your hips and knees flexed to 90 degrees and your feet resting on a chair or wall. Position your core in neutral. Now, take a breath in and see where the air goes. Do you feel your chest or abdomen expand more?

If it is mostly your chest, you need to work on this. Position one hand on your chest and the other hand on your stomach. Focus on breathing that moves the hand on your stomach. Your hand on your chest should remain relatively still. If this is challenging, try applying light pressure to the hand on your chest; this will help to encourage less rise and fall of the chest. Focus on breathing into your hand on your stomach and lightly pressing down with your hand on your chest. Think of the top hand as an elephant that is standing on you, limiting your ability to breathe in air. Now, breathe in through your nose, and exhale through your mouth. Work on this until the major-

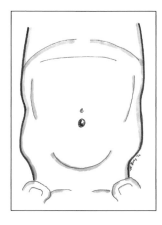

Good breathing pattern with rounded tire-like abdomen.

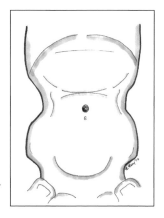

Poor breathing pattern with hourglass effect.

ity of the breath is coming from movement in the abdomen, moving your lower hand.

After you can control this well, take both hands and place them on the sides of your abdomen. Continue to breathe in the same pattern as above, focusing not only on the rise and fall of the abdomen but also the expansion into your hands laterally. We want the expansion of your core to occur circumferentially. To help with this, picture an inner tube that you are trying to fill in all directions. If the air does not fill in all directions, you will have what is known as the hourglass syndrome. This is not efficient.

When you have mastered a good circumferential diaphragmatic breath, work on controlling this in more challenging positions.

Progression of Breathing Positions:

1. On your back with feet supported, hips and knees at 90 degrees.
2. On your back with knees bent and feet flat on the ground.
3. On all fours, hands and knees.
4. On your back with legs flat.
5. Seated on low step with back slightly rounded.
6. Standing.
7. During your core stability exercises.

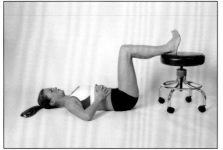

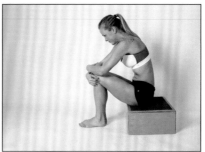

Breathing position number 1.   **Breathing position number 5.**

Breathing and Posture

Now that we have gone over neutral core and breathing, let's apply this to posture. In this case, we are not talking about posture during daily activities, but during core exercises and running. We will discuss the influence of daily postures on our running later.

The foundation of your posture for exercise is rooted deeply in your core position and breathing posture. If you have this controlled, the rest should be fairly easy.

Start with your chest and shoulder position. Your shoulders should be lightly pulled backward and depressed down.

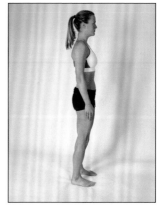

Standing posture with good alignment of head, shoulders, core neutral, knees, and feet.

This should not feel forced but rather like a light retraction opening your chest and relaxing the tops of your shoulders and neck. To help with shoulder posture, try performing the following two exercises occasionally as part of your core routine.

No Money

Sit or stand with a neutral core. Place a small resistance band in or around your hands. Your thumbs should be oriented upward or out to the side. Now, lightly pinch your shoulder blades together while you draw your hands apart. Picture the movement initiating more from your shoulders than your arms. When your hands are apart, perform three relaxed diaphragm breaths and then return. Perform three sets of three to

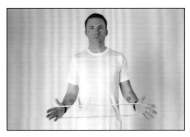

No Money.

five repetitions, holding each for three breaths as a movement preparation exercise for your core routine.

Y Wall Slide

Stand facing a wall. Stagger your legs slightly with one in front of the other like you are running. Set your core into a neutral position and make sure to hold it. Now, with your forearms and hands on the wall, thumbs facing you, slide your forearms up the wall in a "Y" motion, getting wider as you go. Focus on keeping your shoulders down and slightly back as you slide upward. Stop sliding them if your shoulders begin to hike upward. Perform three sets of three to five repetitions, holding each for three breaths. When you can control this movement well, add a slight lift off the wall with your hands when you are at the top of your arm raise. You can also make this more challenging by using a light resistance band around your hands and performing the same motion.

Now that your shoulders are in the correct position, let's look even higher up the chain. Your head should be in line with your eyes facing forward. If you're doing an exercise that is vertical, such as kneeling or standing, pretend that you have a book sitting

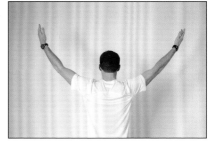

Y Wall Slide.

on top of your head that you do not want to fall off. Finally, when standing, your weight should be evenly distributed between the front and back of your foot. Most tend to stand with excess weight in their heels. This does not center your mass well through your feet. By aligning in the correct posture, your body will be well-centered, which will help with optimal stability.

Keep the parameters of this chapter in mind as you go through the next three chapters. The material here will serve as the foundation for many of the exercises that you will be performing. With this quality in mind, you will maximize benefit from your time spent conditioning your core. Now, let's take a look at core-specific flexibility and mobility.

Chapter 7

Core Specific Mobility and Flexibility

Let me guess: You saw the word "flexibility" and almost skipped this chapter. I get it, runners do not like this stuff, myself included. Anything that takes precious time away from our running is not worth it, right? Well, let's turn the tables the other way. What if we all spent a little more time on flexibility and mobility and in return we were able to run an extra mile or even an extra day next week? Would that be worth it? What if the tradeoff was to be injury-free? This would be hard to argue against.

The majority of runners I treat do not spend time on flexibility and the other necessary maintenance needed for healthy running. It's a little funny how many runners come in the door and say, "I know I should be doing more, but I just can't get myself to do it." Well, now is the time to prioritize your conditioning for running, especially if you had low scores on the mobility and flexibility tests in the self-assessment. Regardless, this chapter is essential for core maintenance.

Flexibility is defined as the length of a muscle or group of muscles that cross the joints to induce a bending movement or motion. It's how far you can stretch a muscle. Mobility, on the other hand, is the ability to move freely and easily. This is about how supple the actual muscle is. Flexibility and mobility combine to create freedom of movement. The more your tissues are able to move with ease, the higher the quality of movement. Mobility is the best foundation for a runner. Without free motion, strength is nothing.

Picture a blob of Silly Putty. You first take it out of the container and it feels like a rock. You might be strong, but it will not come apart easily and if it does, it will achieve its maximum length quickly and even rip in half. However, if you play with the Silly Putty in your hands for a few minutes, it will warm up and soften. With little strength, you will be able to pull the putty apart and stretch it quite a distance before it breaks.

Silly Putty is just like the softer tissues in your body. They also have a maximum length to which they can stretch. This length is something that can be improved, but it will take some time. You need to focus on soft-tissue mobility, flexibility, and posture. Posture has a lot to do with flexibility. Picture sitting in a chair with your hips flexed all day long. Your hip flexors become tight. If you stretch for a few minutes, is it going to help? If you spend a few minutes a day trying to stretch but then hours of the day in postures or positions where muscles are tightening, the odds of improving flexibility are not in your favor. We will look more at the posture component in Chapter 10. First, let's look at how to perform core-specific soft-tissue mobility and flexibility exercises.

Soft-Tissue Mobility

One of the ways you can improve overall mobility and freedom of movement is through self-administering soft-tissue mobility, otherwise known as myofascial release (MFR). MFR is designed to improve tissue warmth and overall mobility, similar to what happened with the Silly Putty above. Soft-tissue mobility will serve you best if you perform it pre- and post-running.

MFR is fairly simple to perform using your hands, a small ball such as a tennis or lacrosse ball, a rolling pin or stick, or a foam roller.

Select your tool based on the area you are working on. You'll apply pressure to the tissue, followed by a multidirectional massage. MFR entails constant self-assessment. Begin the self-massage with larger, sweeping motions, paying close attention to areas that are tighter or sorer. After you finish scanning the area, focus on the spots that have more restriction. They should loosen as you roll over them. After you have worked each of the smaller spots, finish with a few larger sweeps again of the whole area.

The length of the treatment will vary based on how restricted body parts are. This can change from day to day. For example, you may find that you are tighter in the morning or the day after an interval workout. I recommend performing a thirty-second scan of each of the following areas before running most days, as well as after on longer distance days, after harder workouts, during periods of higher mileage, or when peaking for competition. It should only take a few minutes. If you have a history of troublesome spots or notice tightness, you should spend an extra thirty seconds on that area. After performing this routine on a few occasions, you will likely find areas that you need to focus on regularly and others you can trim from your routine.

Follow this routine:

Adductors

The foam roller works best for this. You can also select the stick or ball if you need to focus your pressure deeper. Lie on your side with the leg you plan to roll on top of the roller. Perform an up-and-down motion using your arms and lower leg to help guide the movement, extending from the inner groin to just above the inside of your knee.

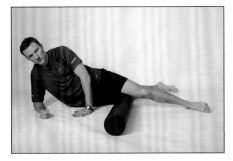

Adductor foam rolling.

Hip Flexors

Use a lacrosse ball for this first. If the pressure is too much, consider a larger ball, such as a softball, or a softer ball, like a tennis ball. If this is still too much pressure, a foam roller may be used on the lower end of the muscle.

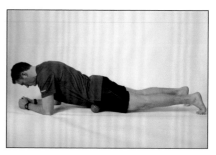
Hip flexor ball rolling.

Lie on your stomach, placing the ball just to the inside of the hip pointer on the front of the hip. Roll up and down, keeping the ball close to the bone. You will be able to roll the lower attachment of the muscle better; it is found just below the bone, wrapping slightly to the inside of the femur.

Quadriceps

The foam roller will work best. Lie on your stomach, placing both legs on top of the foam roller. Roll up and down from just below the front of the hip to the top of the knee. Remember that the quadriceps is a large muscle; therefore,

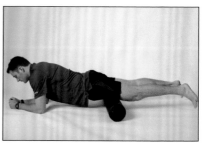
Quadriceps foam rolling.

rolling the outer, middle, and inner front portions of the thigh is important. It is easy to perform this on both legs at one time as long as the level of pressure is adequate. If the pressure is not firm enough, you may need to focus on one leg at a time. You can also use a firmer foam roller or a rolling pin/stick.

Tensor Fascia Latae (TFL)/Iliotibial Band (IT band)

Everyone's favorite: the dreaded IT band. Given that the muscle belly is short and the tendon is long, soft-tissue mobility often is more effective than stretching for this. The foam roller will work best.

Focus on the TFL first. Lie on your stomach with your body rolled slightly to the outside. Roll up and down from the hip pointer to the bone on the outer hip. Second, roll on the IT band by lying on your side with the down leg on top of the roller. Roll up and down from the outer hip bone to the top of the knee.

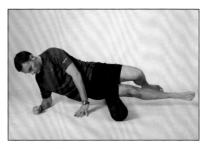

IT band foam rolling.

Gluteus Medius and Outer Hip

Use the foam roller. Lie on your side with the leg you're going to roll on the bottom and the roller between the outer hip bone and hip crest. Cross your top leg and place this foot on the ground to help guide the movement. Perform a small up-and-down rolling motion between the outer hip bone and the top hip crest.

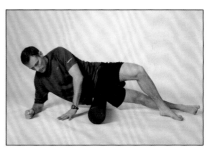

Gluteus medius and outer hip foam rolling.

Gluteus Maximus

The foam roller or ball may be best, depending on the depth that you are trying to achieve. Start by sitting on top of the foam roller and roll over each glute. This likely will not be enough pressure. To increase the pressure, shift your weight to one side and roll one glute at a time. Roll up and down, from the sit bone to the top of the hip. To increase pressure, bend the knee upward or use a ball instead.

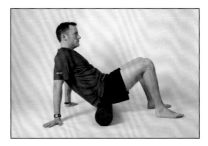

Gluteus maximus foam rolling.

Piriformis and Hip Rotators

Use the foam roller or a ball. Sit in a similar fashion to the above, but with the leg on the side to be rolled on top of the opposite knee. This crossed-leg position will help expose the piriformis and hip rotators. Roll

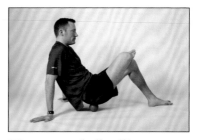

Hip rotators ball rolling.

up and down and side to side on this area.

Hamstring

The stick or ball usually works best for this. The foam roller is typically not able to provide adequate pressure. Roll up and down, from the top of the back of the knee to the bone that you sit on. If you have had symptoms close to the sit bone, focus pressure there in a back-and-

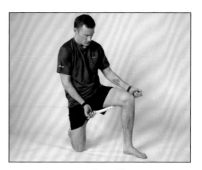

Hamstring stick rolling.

forth direction. Use a ball to achieve an appropriate depth.

Lower Back Soft Tissue

Use a foam roller to focus on the softer tissue on either side of the spine of the lower back. Perform this on your back with your weight shifted to one side. Roll up and down from your hip crest to your rib cage. Placing the arm overhead

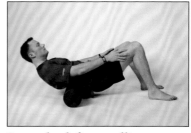

Lower back foam rolling.

on the side that you are treating will help to expose this tissue. Focus on right and left independently. If the pressure is too much, you can also perform this in a standing position by placing your back against the foam roller on the wall.

Thoracic Spine

It's best to use the foam roller. Lie on your back with the roller placed horizontally across your thoracic spine or upper back. Cross your arms across your chest to draw your shoulder blades out of the way. Roll

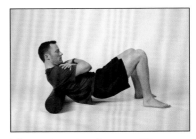

Thoracic spine foam rolling.

up and down, arching your back slightly across the roller as you go. To increase pressure, two tennis balls can be taped together to make a peanut-shaped object. Roll on this in the same fashion that you would on the foam roll.

Static Stretching

Static stretching refers to a stretch in which a muscle is held at a point for a duration of time. This is the most common kind of stretching for most people. Static stretching is different than MFR because it does not have much purpose before running. The longer holds help with elongation of muscles, but not with warming them up.

Unfortunately, this lengthening of the tissue does not happen as easily or as quickly as most think. Holding a stretch for a minute will likely not allow you to gain much length in the short term. Reserve the majority of your static stretching for after your runs and on days or times of the week when you may not be running. If you do decide to perform these stretches with your running, warm up first. You will achieve more from your stretching if you run ten minutes and then stretch your target areas after.

These are the exercises that may take some time but will reward you with long-term gains. Hold each stretch for thirty to sixty seconds. Start with a lighter hold and ease into a deeper stretch as you go. Perform two to three repetitions on the areas where you are most limited. Make these exercises part of your daily routine. Fit the stretches in when you brush your teeth, take a phone call, or watch TV.

Keep in mind that there are a number of ways to perform each of these stretches. Different positions will work best for different individuals. I have selected the positions best for most runners, but also those that are easy to incorporate into daily activities, because if you can stand to do the stretch, you are more likely to find a time to do it.

Adductors

Stand with your feet wide apart. Perform a lunge-like motion, bending your knee to one side, while focusing on keeping the opposite leg straight and dropping your hip downward slightly on this side. Make sure to maintain a neutral lower spine curvature. You should feel a stretch on the inner thigh of the straight leg.

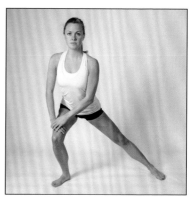

Standing adductor stretch.

Iliopsoas

Kneel with one knee on the ground (a pillow or rolled-up shirt may make this more comfortable) and the opposite knee bent 90 degrees in front of you with that foot on the ground. Tuck your toes underneath on the back foot, so that your foot is vertical. The next step is key to achieving the optimal position. Tilt your pelvis underneath you so

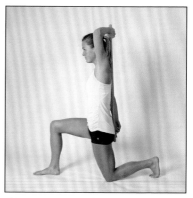

Iliopsoas stretch using stick on back.

that your lower back is in a neutral position. To do this, imagine your breathing posture. Tightening your glutes and stomach will also help. While holding this position, shift your hips forward while maintaining a vertical torso position. You should feel a stretch in the front of the hip whose knee is on the ground. You may also feel this down your thigh. You should not have discomfort in your back—if you do, focus more on the hip position while you move forward. Holding a stick vertically on your back can help keep you in the correct position. Focus on maintaining the gap between the stick and your back as you move forward.

Rectus Femoris/Iliopsoas

Stand facing away from a chair. Bend one knee and place this leg behind you with that foot on the chair. Focus again here on a neutral spine, like you did for your hip flexor in the previous stretch. Shift your hips forward and then lower them slowly by bending your knee that is on the ground. You should feel a stretch in the front of the hip and thigh on the leg that is bent. If not, you may need to use a higher object such as a table or the back of a bench.

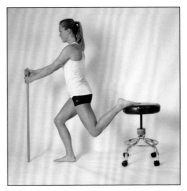

Rectus femoris/iliopsoas standing stretch.

TFL/IT Band—Standing Banana

As mentioned in the soft-tissue mobility section, the IT band is loosened better through MFR. This stretch will isolate the TFL portion; therefore, you should feel this more in the front outer hip. Stand with your legs crossed and the stretching leg in the back with the foot turned inward.

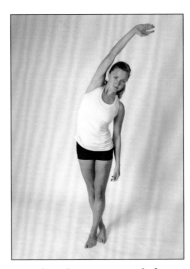

Standing banana stretch for TFL/IT band.

Reach overhead with your arm on the same side as the stretching leg while moving your hips laterally, toward the non-stretching foot. Focus on keeping most of your weight on the side that is being stretched.

Hamstring—Toe Touch

Stand on one leg, placing the other about a foot in front. Straighten the lead leg and raise your foot upward. Reach down toward your toes with both hands, leaning from your hips. Make sure that your back remains straight and does not arch. It is

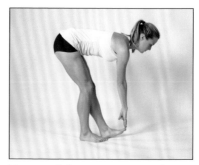

Toe touch hamstring stretch.

more important that your back remains flat. Do not sacrifice a bend in your back to touch your toes.

A nice alternative to the toe touch is an active hamstring kick-up. To perform this, while on your back, raise one leg up, grabbing with both hands behind your knee. Keep your opposite leg flat on the ground. Now, straighten the knee of the leg that is in the air until you feel a stretch in the hamstring. Because of the active component of this stretch, it does not follow the normal static stretching hold and repetition parameters. Instead, hold for ten seconds and perform ten repetitions per side.

Gluteus Maximus and Gluteus Medius

Lie on your back. Pull one knee toward your chest, keeping the other leg straight and flat on the ground. This will isolate the gluteus maximus on the side that is bent, meaning that you should feel a stretch in your butt. To focus more

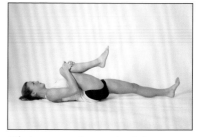

Gluteus maximus stretch.

on the gluteus medius, keep the hip and knee bent, pulling the leg across the body. You should feel this on the outer hip, but through the butt as well.

Piriformis and Hip Rotators—Modified Pigeon

This can be performed stand-ing or lying on your stomach. For the standing position, rotate your leg across your body so that your knee is bent and then place this leg on top of a table. Now, lean forward, rotating the oppo-site shoulder toward your knee in front. You should feel a stretch

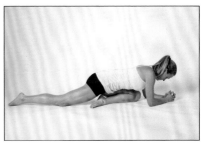

Pigeon stretch for piriformis and hip rotators.

deep in your glute region. If not, the stomach position may be bet-ter for you because it often leads to a deeper stretch. This will be performed similarly by lying on your stomach with one leg bent and rotated underneath you. The opposite leg should be straight behind you. Again, lower the opposite shoulder toward the bent knee until a stretch is felt.

Thoracic Spine Rotation

Lie on one side with your top knee bent and raised in front of you higher than your hip. Place the top leg on top of a foam roller or medicine ball to keep it ele-vated off the ground. Hold this knee with the arm that is on the ground. Now rotate backward through your shoulders, reaching

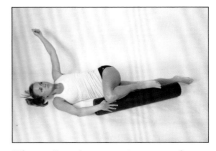

Thoracic spine rotation stretch using foam roller.

behind you with the top arm. Focus on moving your shoulders as far as you're able. Stop when you feel a stretch in your back. At this point, perform multiple breaths, focusing on rotating slightly more during each exhale.

Lumbar and Thoracic Spine—Child's Pose

Kneel on the ground with both knees and then sit back on your heels. If you have knee discomfort, put a pillow or rolled towel on your heels and sit on it to keep your knees from bending as far. Lean forward so that your arms are on the ground in front of you. Keep your hips seated on your heels or

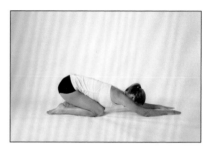

Child's pose stretch for lumbar and thoracic spine.

the pillow. Perform multiple breaths, reaching forward while pressing your shoulders to the ground on each exhale. Focus also on tucking your pelvis and rounding your lower back.

Dynamic Stretching

These are stretches that require movement. They are held for five seconds or less and are designed to increase blood flow, along with soft-tissue mobility. Dynamic stretching can be performed before running. You can also do them during running, if you are taking a break between intervals or you have an onset of tightness during a run. Think of these as warm-up or muscle preparation exercises to achieve short-term gains. They are not designed to increase flexibility in a muscle in the long term. Pay specific attention to the overall control of your body. You will achieve more from each exercise by focusing on quality of core control and balance during each one.

When you warm up, remember "the big eight for twenty-five." This means that there are eight dynamic stretches to do before you run as a dynamic core warm-up. With the exception of the leg swings, perform these in a walking fashion for twenty-five feet each. For example, perform the stretch on one side, take a step, and then perform the stretch on the other. After you have completed a lap, progress to the next stretch. The leg swings are an exception—perform these in place, completing twenty-five repetitions.

World's Greatest Stretch—Hip Flexor, Glute, Spine

While standing, take a big lunge forward while keeping both of your feet straight ahead. Lower your hips to the ground and place both hands down to the inside of the lead foot. Lift the hand that is closest to the front foot and rotate your torso away from it while reaching with this arm. You should feel a stretch in the front of the hip of the back leg. You may also feel

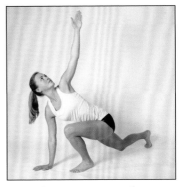

World's greatest stretch.

a stretch in the glute and hamstring of the lead leg as well as your back. Hold this position for three to five seconds and then stand up and repeat on the other side. To get a little more from this stretch, incorporate a calf stretch by keeping the heel down when you first step forward; after this, go into the big lunge and proceed with the rest of the motion.

Standing Superman Reach—Quad, Hip Flexor, Hamstring

While standing, bend one knee, grabbing your foot behind you. Pull this leg backward slightly while focusing on maintaining a neutral spine. You should start to feel a stretch in the front of your hip and thigh. Now

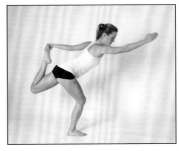

Standing Superman reach stretch.

bend forward from your hips, reaching with the opposite arm in front. This will start to stretch the hamstring of the leg that is on the ground. Hold this position for three to five seconds, stand up, take a step forward, and repeat on the other side.

Cross-Body Knee Grab—Glute, Hip Rotators

While standing, bend your knee, lift it in front, then grab the ankle with the opposite hand and place the other hand on the outer knee. Lift your leg up and across your body. Use your hands to direct your knee to the opposite shoulder. You should feel a stretch through your outer hip and glute region. Hold for three to five seconds, then step forward and repeat on the opposite side.

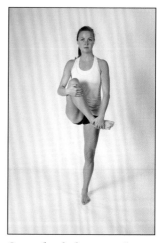

Cross-body knee-grab stretch.

Knee to Chest—Glute, Hip Flexor

While standing, pull one knee up to your chest and hold for three to five seconds. You should feel a stretch in your glute. Release this side and take a step forward. Repeat on the other side. If this is well-controlled, you can add a balance component by performing a small heel raise with each step.

Frankensteins—Hamstring

Standing tall, perform a straight leg kick forward with one leg. Reach forward with your opposite hand. Try to make your foot and hand land in the midline

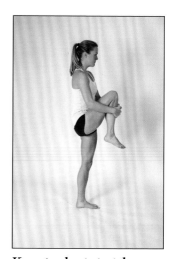

Knee to chest stretch.

of your body. Keep your torso tall and do not worry if they are not able to touch each other. Alternate kicks on each side while walking forward. These should be performed slowly, holding the leg in the up position for a controlled one second with each repetition. You should feel light tension in your hamstring.

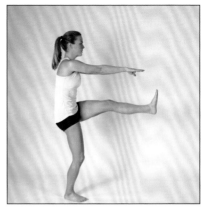

Frankenstein stretch.

Alternating Toe Touches—Hamstring, Calf, Spine

Step forward with one leg about twelve inches, placing your heel on the ground while your foot is pointing upward as much as possible. Keep your knee straight and reach down, bending from your hips, with the opposite hand toward your toes and grab them

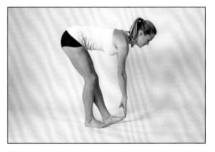

Alternating toe touch stretch.

if you can. Make sure that your back stays flat and does not round through the lumbar spine. You should feel a stretch in the back of the lead leg. Hold this position for three to five seconds, stand back up, take a step, and repeat on the other side. You can add a spinal rotation stretch by reaching your hand on the side of the forward leg toward the ceiling, allowing your torso to rotate along with your arm.

Leg Swings Forward/Backward—Hamstring, Hip

Stand next to something you are able to hold on to for balance. Bend one knee slightly and keep this foot on the ground. Perform a forward/backward leg swing in each direction, making sure to focus on control of your core. Allow only minimal movement in your hips

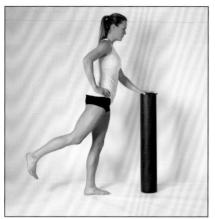
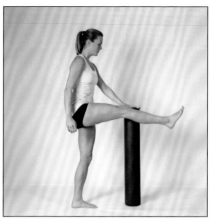

Forward/backward leg swing start position.   **Forward/backward leg swing finish position.**

and lower back. You should feel slight tension in the front and back of your hip and leg with each swing. Start with a smaller amplitude swing and increase as you go. Perform twenty-five repetitions on each side.

Leg Swings Sideways—Abductors/Adductors

Stand facing something that you are able to hold on to for balance. Bend one knee slightly and keep this foot on the ground. Perform

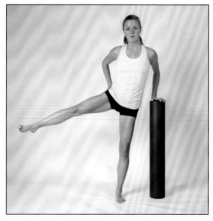
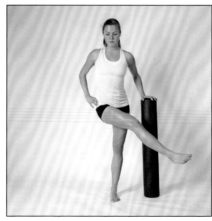

Sideways leg swing start position.   **Sideways leg swing finish position.**

a side-to-side leg swing in front of you with the opposite leg. Keep your core engaged during this but allow rotation in your hips and spine to occur. You should feel slight tension in the inner thigh and outer hip with each swing. Again, start with a smaller amplitude swing and increase as you go. Perform twenty-five repetitions on each side.

Remember that everyone's routine should be tailored specifically to his or her needs. If you notice muscles requiring more attention, they should be placed higher in your priorities. Areas that do not seem to be tight should be placed lower on the list, to be checked less frequently.

Now, let's move on to core stability and strengthening.

Chapter 8
Core Stabilization and Strength

When you think of core strength, what is the first exercise that comes to mind? Is it a crunch or a sit-up? For years, these have been a staple in school gym classes, military conditioning, and many gym routines. Is this really a beneficial exercise?

Think about what happens as you do a sit-up: Your abdominal musculature contracts, flexing your stomach region, causing you to bend forward, hinging through the back. Now, think about running. How often do you bend this way during a run? Hopefully never. So, if this motion is not even a part of running, why perform it? Crunches and sit-ups will help improve strength of an isolated region that is not specific to a runner. Think back to Chapter 2 and the discussion of what the core is doing when you run. For the most part, you are moving through the hips and stabilizing through the rest of your core.

So, what is the difference between core stability and strength? These terms are often used interchangeably, but it is important to recognize that they are different. Strength refers to the ability to produce a given force, whereas stability refers to the ability to control those forces. Think of lifting weights in the gym. You may be able to perform a 200-pound bench press using a machine with ease. However, if you try to bench press the same weight but split it into

100-pound dumbbells, you may not be able to do it. You have the strength to press the 200 pounds but you may not have the ability to stabilize and control it, making the individual weights much harder. For a runner, strength is important for the foundation of the core but it is truly expressed as stability as you run.

A runner came into my clinic and said his glutes were hibernating. I love this description because it is quite accurate for many of us. Many runners have done extensive work on their glutes, hips, and core, but neither their form nor their level of pain changes. That's because strengthening is never connected to movement. If something is hibernating, strengthening wakes it up short-term—while you are doing the exercise—but it goes right back to sleep afterward. To see improvement, you need to wake the muscle up and then use it. First, you want to activate the muscle, then strengthen it, and finally use it through stabilization or movement. This multistep process is the key to not only improving strength, but also maintaining a higher level for years to come.

This chapter will go through multiple core exercises for strength and also stabilization specific to runners. Each exercise has a tiered progression ranging from beginner (B), to intermediate (I), advanced (A), and Expert (E) levels. Pay close attention to technique during each exercise. Form is more important than duration or repetition. Refer to the discussion on breathing and posture in Chapter 6. If you focus on the quality of the exercises, you will maximize the benefit from each.

Start with the "Beginner" form of each exercise and work your way through the rankings based on your ability to perform them. Also, start with the lower set and repetition ranges and slowly advance them as well. When you can perform an exercise with higher sets and repetitions, consider challenging yourself through added resistance or advancing to the next exercise. Based on your scoring of Part C of Chapter 5, the core-stabilization component, you may find that you need to spend more time on the beginner-level exercises or progress faster.

The core exercises that we are going to focus on in this chapter can be done in your home workout space with minimal equipment. You will need a resistance band that is either formed or tied in a loop. These come in varying resistances. If you do need to purchase bands, look for a pack that has different levels of resistance so that you can progress to the harder levels as your strength improves. You will also need a longer resistance band that is not tied. These come with handles but they are not necessary. You can just use a long piece of flat resistance band or tubing. Some of the exercises will also require a light set of dumbbells, a medicine ball, a physio ball, and a kettlebell. Don't rush out and buy everything—get creative in the beginning, such as using a filled water bottle to mimic the dumbbells or a small grocery bag with some rocks in it to replicate the kettlebell. As you get into your routine, you will figure out which equipment and resistances will work best for your routine.

Perform these exercises with your shoes off so that you can focus more on what your feet are doing. When performing exercises with your feet planted on the ground, splay your toes as much as possible and press the pads of your toes into the ground. By increasing activation of the foot and lower leg, overall stabilization and ground-to-body feedback will improve. Now, let's get that core stabilized and strong.

Core Strength Exercises

Clamshell Progression:

The standard clamshell focuses on strengthening the external rotators of the hip. Performing the opposite motion or reverse clamshell, you will isolate the internal rotators of the hip. Perform two to four sets of twenty to twenty-five repetitions. Increase the intensity of the resistance band as tolerated. If you are not able to control the motion, start without resistance and progress to using bands as you improve. These exercises should be felt in your outer and deeper hip, as well as your glute.

Clamshell (B)

Start on one side with a band around your knees. Bend your knees to approximately 90 degrees with your knees lying in front of you at the level of your hips. Take your top hand and press it into the floor, so that your core tightens. Now, perform a

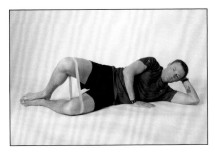

Clamshell.

clamshell motion by opening your knees while keeping your feet together. Squeeze your outer hip and glute. Perform this slowly, keeping your top hip in place and slightly rolled forward.

Reverse Clamshell (B)

The reverse clamshell focuses more on the internal rotators of the hip, but with some underlying stability and strength from the other muscles. Start with the same body and hand position as the clamshell. This time the band will be around your ankles. Raise

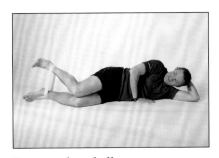

Reverse clamshell.

your top foot while keeping your knees and hips in place.

Super Clamshell (A)

Start in a similar position to the clamshell with your knees bent to 90 degrees but a little lower than the level of your hips. Elevate into a side plank on your elbow and knee. Reach to the ceiling with your top hand and maintain this position. Make sure your core is engaged, and perform the clamshell motion slowly from this position.

Super Duper Clamshell (E)

Start in your super clamshell position on your side, then raise up to a side plank. To do this, you will elevate both knees and hips off the ground so that you are supported from your feet and forearm. From here, perform a clamshell motion by opening both legs, drawing the bottom leg down and the top leg up.

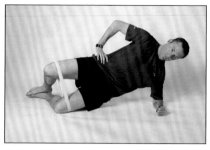

Super clamshell.

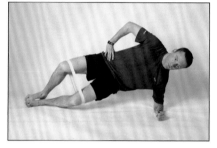

Super duper clamshell.

Resistance-Band Walks:

Resistance-band walks are an excellent way to strengthen the hip muscles and work on core control. Focus on the neutral core position that you learned in Chapter 6 to make sure the stability component is not forgotten. Perform two to four sets of a twenty-foot distance. Increase the intensity of the resistance band as tolerated. You can also increase difficulty and muscle activation by moving the band from your knees to your ankles, and around your feet (except on the Tandem Walk).

Sideways Walk (B)

From a standing position with a band on, perform a mini squat by bending your knees and sticking your butt out slightly. Maintain this position along with neutral core. Perform small side steps, about eight

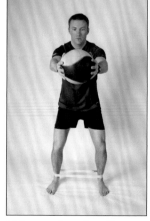

Sideways band walk.

to twelve inches, maintaining tension on the band at all times. This should be done slowly with your feet and knees pointing straight ahead. Have one leg lead and then switch directions to have the other leg lead.

Monster Walk (I)

Assume the same starting position, with the band, as the side step, but face forward and keep your feet together. Take a forward diagonal step outward. Bring your trail leg to meet this one briefly; then your trail leg will step forward and diagonally in the other direction. Alternate diagonal steps slowly while maintaining tension in the band. Perform this first by walking forward and then backward.

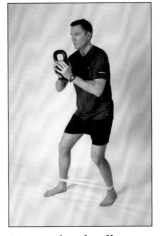

Monster band walk.

Retro Walk "Train Tracks" (I)

This exercise will also be performed in the same position as above with the band, but with your feet starting just wider than shoulder-width. You will maintain this wide stance throughout. Walk backward at a steady pace, performing quick little steps. Pretend that your feet are on train tracks so that they keep the wider width and stay pointing straight as you move.

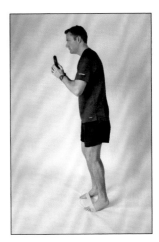

Retro band walk. "Train tracks."

Tandem Walk (A)

For this exercise, keep your knees almost straight but not locked. Remember, the band can go around your knees or ankles for more challenge, but don't place it around your feet for this exercise. Place one foot in front of the other to start. Pick a line on the ground and walk this like you are walking a tightrope. With each step, maintain the tension on the band by taking a big swooping step out and around. Make sure your core is tight and you are able to control your balance. Go forward and then backward.

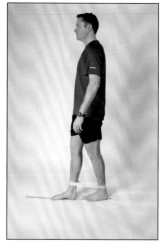

Tandem band walk.

Leg Raises/Kicks:

Straight leg raises can be performed on your back, sides, and stomach to isolate muscles on all sides of your hip. Maintain an engaged core and keep the leg straight by tightening your thigh and pulling back slightly on your foot. Perform two to four sets of fifteen to twenty-five repetitions. Increase the intensity by adding weight to your ankle as tolerated. These can also be performed in a standing position known as "Steamboats." For this, apply resistance through a band tied to a firm object low to the ground. Similar sets and repetitions should be followed.

Three-Way Leg Raises (B)

The three leg raises will be performed from each of your sides and your back. Your thigh should be held tight and your knee straight. Keep your foot pointing in the direction that your torso is facing. Lift your leg about one foot off the ground, then slowly lower. For the side leg raises, press your top hand into the ground to help core activation. During the leg raise on your back, press both arms downward.

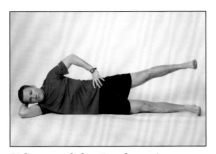

Sideways abduction leg raise.

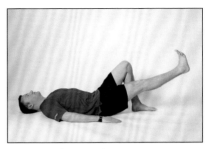

Forward flexion leg raise.

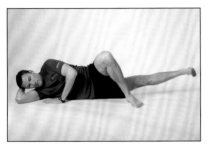

Inside adduction leg raise.

Donkey Kick (B)

The donkey kick is the fourth direction for your leg raise, isolating the gluteus maximus. Get down on all fours. Hold your core tight. Elevate the working leg in the air behind you with your knee bent to 90 degrees. Press your foot toward the ceil-

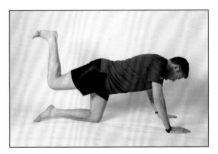

Donkey kick.

ing while keeping your ankle flexed to 90 degrees by squeezing your glute, and then slowly lower. Do not overarch your back as you kick up. Keep your head relaxed and in line with your torso.

Four-Way Standing Leg Raise "Steamboats" (I)

These four exercises will be performed from the standing position. You will perform a leg raise in four different directions: forward, inward across your body, backward, and outward to the side. Place a band around one leg with the other end tied firmly on a leg of a table. For the first position, face away from the table. Balance on the

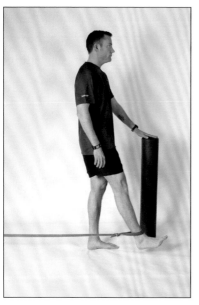

Forward flexion steamboat.

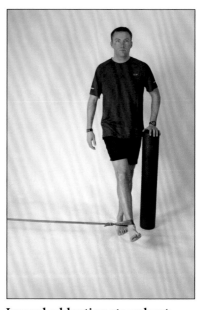

Inward adduction steamboat.

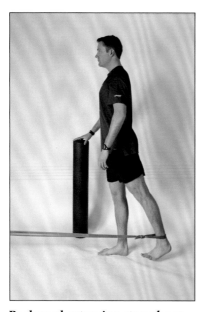

Backward extension steamboat.

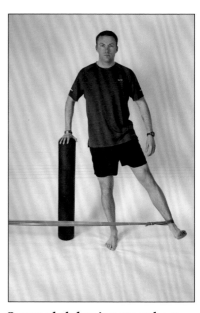

Outward abduction steamboat.

opposite leg with your knee slightly bent. Stretch the band about one foot in front of you, then slowly return it to the starting position. After you have completed a set, rotate your body a quarter turn in either direction and then perform a raise in that direction against the resistance of the band. Continue this pattern until you have pulled the band in all four directions. You can do lower repetitions at a slower pace, or experiment with faster-paced, higher repetitions for variation.

Side-Lying Runner (I)

This is a bonus exercise. It works similar muscles as the sideways leg raise and standing outward kick steamboat. I like this because it works the outer hip in a similar way as running does. From a sideways lying position, tighten your core (pressing the top hand

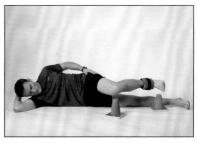

Side-lying runner.

into the ground will again help). Perform a circular running stride motion with the top leg. Make sure that your leg stays parallel to the ground and does not drop.

Squat Progression:

Squatting is an essential movement for a runner because running is consecutive repetitions of single-leg squats. Squats strengthen the legs by focusing on quadriceps and gluteals. Pay close attention to foot and knee alignment—the feet and knees should point straight ahead, as they would when you run. Many runners have the tendency to allow their knees to cave inward when they squat, which is not good form. Also, be sure to control your pelvis and lumbar spine in a neutral position throughout. If you need a refresher on this position, refer back to Chapter 6. Perform two or three sets of ten to fifteen repetitions. Increase the intensity by adding weight. Consider placing a band at your knees. By keeping tension on the band, it will help to cue further core stabilization and help prevent your knees from caving inward. You can further challenge yourself with single-leg squats on an uneven surface, like a small cushion.

Two-Leg (B)

Stand with your feet just wider than shoulder width and your feet pointing straight ahead. Initiate the squatting motion by dropping your hips backward like you are sitting into a chair. Allow your knees to move forward but not much farther than your toes. Keep your head and chest upright. Pressing your hands in front of you as you go lower can help with this. During the movement, make sure your core is engaged, feet and knees are pointing forward, and your back is straight (but not vertical). To initiate the return to standing,

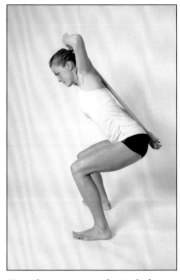

Two-leg squat with stick for spine alignment.

squeeze your glutes and push into the ground evenly from your feet. If you are new to the squat pattern, place a broomstick flat on your back extending from your hips, upper back, and head. This will help maintain a straight spine. You can also place a box vertically at your toes to help maintain proper form by keeping your knees from protruding in front of your toes.

Two-Leg Suitcase (I)

The suitcase squat uses the same technique as above. Here, hold resistance in one hand, like a dumbbell or kettlebell. Because the resistance is in only one hand, it will force your core to activate more on the opposite side. Perform a normal squat maintaining a centered body position. Do not let the weight pull you to the side. Perform ten to fifteen repetitions on one side, then switch hands with the resistance and perform ten to fifteen on the other.

One-Leg Step-Down (A)

After you have mastered the two-leg squat, we will work on the single-leg versions. The same technique applies. I prefer to do this off a box or step if available, because it helps guide the depth of your squat. When your foot hits the ground, you have hit the depth that you are aiming for. Increase the height of the step, thus increasing the depth, as you improve. Standing with one leg firmly planted on a box, squat down, reaching the other leg slightly behind you until it touches the ground. Focus on squeezing through the glutes and quad to return to standing. Pay close attention to your knee alignment. If your knee falls inward, clench your outer hip during the movement.

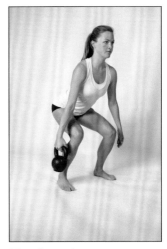

Two-leg suitcase squat.

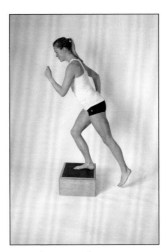

One-leg step down.

One-Leg Suitcase Squat (E)

This exercise is exactly the same as the one above, but with a weight in one hand. Hold the weight on the same side as the squatting leg. This will challenge the opposite side of the core, similar to the stance phase of gait when running. Perform ten to fifteen repetitions on one side and then switch and perform the same on the other.

Romanian Dead Lift (RDL) Progression:

An RDL is an essential exercise in every runner's quiver. It focuses on the development of gluteal and hamstring strength as well as global core stabilization. Most runners are dominant through the quadriceps and need more focus on the muscles in back

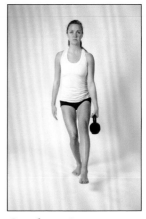

One-leg suitcase squat.

of their legs. It is extremely important to focus on form and technique during this exercise to avoid excessive load on the spine. I recommend having formal instruction from a certified personal trainer, physical therapist, or other exercise specialist before adding resistance. Perform two or three sets of ten to fifteen repetitions. Increase the intensity by adding more resistance through higher weights. As with single-leg squats, increase the challenge of single-leg RDLs by performing them on an unstable surface, like a small pillow.

Two-Leg RDL with Stick Assist (B)

The RDL should first be performed with a non-weighted stick on your back to help with form. Start with a broomstick on your back extending from your hips, upper back, and head. Stand with your feet shoulder-width apart and your knees slightly bent. Initiate a forward bend by reaching your hips backward. Pretend like you are trying to touch something with your glutes a few inches behind you. Focus on maintaining a

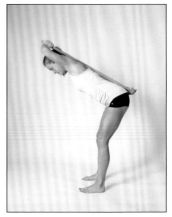

Two-leg RDL using stick to help spine alignment.

straight torso, hinging from your hips and not your spine. Keep the stick on your back touching your head, upper back, and top of the hips at all times. You should also have a small gap between the stick and the lower back at all times. This distance should not change as you perform the movement. Your knees can slightly bend as you go lower but the primary motion should occur through your hip joint. Stop the movement before your back moves or if your hamstrings tighten. Individuals who have poor hamstring flexibility may not be able to go as low. Control is more important than depth here. To return to standing, focus on squeezing your glutes and pressing your hips forward. The lift should be performed through your upper legs and hips, not your back.

Two-Leg Resisted RDL (I)

When you are able to control the RDL movement pattern, add resistance. Start with resistance evenly distributed between your hands, using dumbbells or one barbell or kettlebell using both hands. You can vary this by performing a two-leg RDL with resistance in one hand only. This places more emphasis on rotational trunk control.

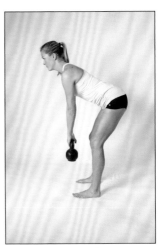

Two-leg resisted RDL.

Single-Leg With or Without Resistance (A/E)

The single-leg RDL is a complex movement pattern that also forces you to balance. Start without resistance. Stand on one leg and perform the same pattern as the two-leg RDL. The opposite leg should be straight and reach behind you as you bend forward. Think about pressing your heel away from you as you go to maintain a straight line through the back leg, your torso, and head through the entire movement. Perform this slowly, making sure that you are balancing and controlling your knee position on your standing leg. Also, keep your hips level. After you can control this without resistance, hold a light weight in your hand on the same side as your raised leg.

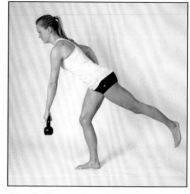

Single-leg resisted RDL.

Airplane (E)

The airplane is an extension of the single-leg RDL. It is quite challenging to integrate many components of strength, stability, and balance. Perform a single-leg RDL as you did in the previous exercise, but with your arms held horizontally out to your sides. Point your thumbs toward your back at all times. When you are at the bottom of your movement pattern, let the fun begin. Slowly perform an upward rotation of your trunk, arms, and extended leg. Think of this like a twisting

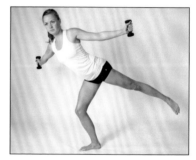

Airplane.

motion occurring from your hip on the side that is on the ground. Your torso will start facing the ground and slowly rotate so that it is on its side. Make sure your trunk, arms, and extended leg all move together, focusing on keeping your hips and shoulders square as you do this. Also, make sure your stance leg does not move as the rest of your body does. Your knee will have the tendency to fall inward, but keep your outer glute tight and do not let this happen. When you have rotated fully, stop, and then lower back to the starting position and finally stand back up. That completes a repetition. You can add dumbbell resistance to your hands as your technique improves.

Nordic Curl (E)

This is a bonus exercise. It is not a deadlift pattern but it isolates the hamstrings. It is performed in an eccentric fashion, which is an area of the running stride that gets many into trouble. This is an easy exercise to perform but places a high degree of load on the hamstring, so it is rated as an expert-level activity

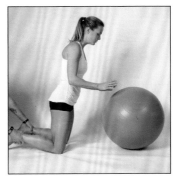

Nordic Curl.

and should be introduced with caution to your routine. Perform two sets of ten repetitions until you see how your body responds to it.

Start by kneeling with both knees on the ground. Have someone hold your ankles firmly or place them under an object that will not move. Keep your core neutral. Have a high object, such as a chair, about one to two feet in front of you to start. You can move the object further as you improve. Slowly lower your torso forward, stopping the movement with your arms. Use your arms to return to the upright posture. When you are able to lower yourself to the chair with good control, find an object that is slightly lower.

Core Stability Exercises

Bridge Progression:

A bridge is designed to improve activation and strength of the gluteals while focusing on stabilization of the core. Pay close attention to control of your pelvis, lumbar spine, and rib cage to maintain a neutral core posture. Keep your arms at your side with your hands flat on the ground. Applying light pressure through your hands into the ground will help to increase core stabilization. Perform two to four sets of ten to fifteen repetitions. Increase the intensity by using a higher-level resistance band as tolerated. A bridge can be made more challenging by using a more unstable ball, such as a smaller medicine ball or something firmer like a basketball.

Two-Leg Bridge (B)

Lie on your back with both knees bent and your feet flat on the ground at shoulder width. Perform a light tuck of your pelvis, making your lower back flat and depressing your lower ribs. Focus on holding this posture. Squeeze your glutes

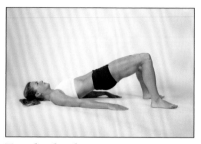

Two-leg bridge.

to lift your hips up while pressing down through your heels. Stop when you feel like you are unable to control your hips. The height is not important with this exercise, so do not try to go too high. When this is well-controlled, add a resistance band to your knees; make sure that your knees stay as wide as your feet. Hold the top position for two to three seconds with each repetition.

Marching Bridge with Band (I)

Perform the same two-leg bridge as above, but pause with your hips in the elevated position. Use a light resistance band around your knees and focus on maintaining the tension on the band during the exercise. Perform slow alternat-

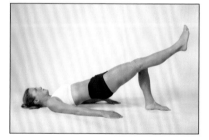

Marching bridge with band.

ing kick-ups by straightening your leg, as though you were marching. Keep your knees in place and make sure your hips stay level.

One-Leg Bridge (A)

To perform a one-leg bridge, elevate one leg to 90 degrees at your hip and knee. The leg will maintain this position during the

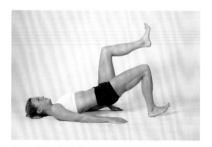

One-leg bridge.

movement. Center the other leg slightly and perform your bridge pattern. Make sure your hips remain level left to right. You can advance this by placing a foam roller under your foot on the down leg. If you want to take one more step, try placing a small medicine ball under the down foot.

One-Leg Bridge with Physio Ball Hamstring Curl (E)

Use a large physio ball. Place one leg straight in front and on top of the ball. The opposite leg is bent at 90 degrees from your hip and knee, like the standard one-leg bridge. Perform a bridge focusing on control of your core. You may need to use your hands to help balance at

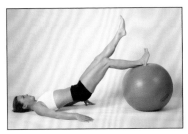

One-leg bridge with physio ball hamstring curl.

first; to do this, place them on the side and apply light pressure into the ground when your hips are elevated, perform a slow roll of the ball toward you, and then out so that your leg is back to the straight starting position. If you are not familiar with the physio ball, try this with two legs on top of the ball and progress to one.

Plank Progression:

The plank position is important in the development of core stabilization. To maximize benefit from a plank, it must be performed with correct technique, keeping the body in a straight line and the core in a neutral position. Controlled breathing is also important. Perform three to five sets of thirty to sixty seconds. Rather than using a timer, consider counting a set by number of breaths. Perform five to ten breaths in a set. Counting breaths forces you to focus more on the control of posture and less on just completing the duration. Quality is imperative!

Plank (B)

To perform a basic elbow plank, lie face down on the floor, with elbows positioned underneath your shoulders. Raise your shoulders and hips so that you are supported from your forearms and feet. Keep your core

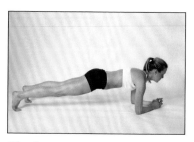

Plank.

engaged by holding your glutes and abdomen tight. Do not let your lower back sag downward, and maintain a straight posture through your ankles, knees, hips, and shoulders. If you are unable to achieve thirty seconds with good control, perform on your hands and feet or elbows and knees. When you are able to hold these positions for thirty to sixty seconds, revert to the elbows-and-feet position.

Foot Walk-Outs (I)

Perform a plank from your elbows and feet like you did in the previous exercise. Slowly walk your feet apart by performing slow alternating steps, about six inches each time. Stop the walk-out when your feet are a comfortable width apart. Focus on squeezing your glute to lift the leg that you are moving. Make sure your lower back does not dip as the leg is in the air. When your feet are apart, slowly walk them back together.

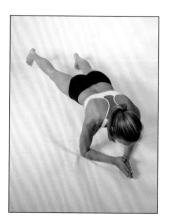

Foot walk-outs.

Ball Plank (A)

For this exercise, you will perform the same plank posture but place your forearms or hands on a physio ball. Start with the ball against a wall to help your

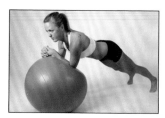

Ball plank.

stability. As you gain control of this, perform the exercise with the ball on an open floor.

Stir the Pots (E)

This is a great variation of the ball plank. Perform a plank with your forearms on the ball. Now perform a small circular motion with your forearms as though you were stirring a pot. Keep your body in place, especially your shoulders, and try to move only through your arms and the ball as you do this. Perform at a variety of speeds and a different number of alternating repetitions each way. You can also add forward and backward and side-to-side movements to increase the fun.

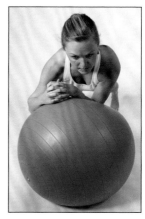

Stir the pots.

Ball Walk-Out (E)

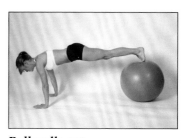

Ball walk-out.

The stomach plank progression finishes with the ball walk-out. Start by lying face down on top of the ball. Roll forward until your hands are on the ground. Slowly walk your hands forward, rolling your torso and then legs over the ball. When your feet are vertical on the ball, pause and then work your way back to the start position. Think of this exercise as a moving plank position from your hands and feet. Maintain a nice straight line through your body during its entirety.

Side Plank Progression:

A side plank is a variation of the standard plank as shown above. It isolates the lateral core. These should be performed with similar posture and breathing in mind. Follow the same three to five sets of thirty to sixty seconds, or count breaths of five to ten in a set.

Side Plank (B)

Lie down on one side with your elbow placed underneath the shoulder and legs stacked. Raise yourself up onto your elbow and forearm, placing your top foot slightly in front of the bottom foot, keeping your body straight and your hips up. Make sure your hips do not sag.

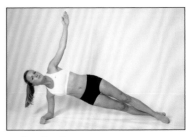

Side plank.

Raise your top hand toward the ceiling during. As always, make sure your core is held tight. If you are unable to hold this position for thirty seconds, start by performing from your forearm and knee. When you are able to hold for thirty to sixty seconds, return to the side plank from your feet.

Side Plank with Resisted Lowering (I)

Here you will perform the same side plank as above while holding a dumbbell in the hand that is in the air. Slowly raise and lower the weight, leading with the thumb in both directions.

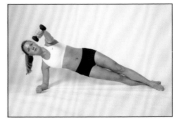

Side plank with resisted lowering.

Side Plank Rotations (A)

Start in a side plank from your forearm and feet. Keep your top foot in front of the bottom. Rotate your body forward toward the top leg that is in front and roll into a basic stomach plank on your

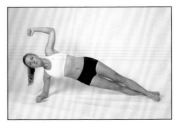

Side plank rotation start position before lowering to elbow plank.

forearms, then roll to a side plank on the opposite side. When you are in this position, remember to keep your top leg positioned in front. Slowly rotate back and forth from side to side, pausing briefly in the regular plank position when face down between each rotation.

Quadruped or All-Fours Progression:

Quadruped is another name for a hands-and-knees position or on all fours. This position helps to tuck the sacrum and round the pelvis underneath you. It is designed for core stabilization, incorporating rotational stability, which is key for a runner. It is a good exercise to focus on early if you are a novice with core stability training. Be mindful during these that your back is not dipped toward the ground and rather only slightly dipped or almost flat. Perform two to four sets of ten to fifteen repetitions per side. As an alternative to counting the number of repetitions, consider counting by breaths as you did with a plank. Perform a set of three to five repetitions per side, holding the position for three to five breaths each time. You can further challenge yourself by narrowing your hands and knee or foot width.

Leg Reach (B)

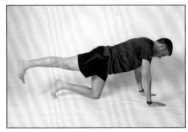

Leg reach in quadruped.

Start on your hands and knees with your head in line with your torso and held in a relaxed position. Keep your core tight with minimal sag in your lower back throughout. Slowly perform alternating backward leg reaches with each leg. Focus on extending your leg straight behind you, reaching backward through your heel and not just lifting up. Control your torso movement left and right during this. A good cue to help with core control is to place a water bottle or foam roller on your back during this progression.

Alternating Arm and Leg Reach or "Bird Dog" (I)

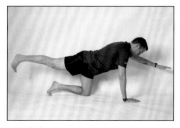

Bird dog.

Perform the first position with the alternating leg reaches while simultaneously performing opposite arm reaches. You can perform this two ways: alternate opposite arms and legs back and forth, or perform multiple reps with one leg and the opposite arm in a row and then switch to the other arm and leg and repeat. If you are doing more than one repetition in a row, slowly lower your elbow to knee between each while still in the air and then return to the extended position. As this gets easier, try moving your hands and knees closer together. An advanced version of this can be done by holding the extended position and slowly drawing six-inch box motions in the air with your foot and hand at the same time. The key is controlling your core as you make the small motions in the air.

Bear Crawl (E)

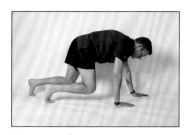

Bear crawl.

Start on all fours and round your back slightly toward the ceiling. Raise your knees off the ground slightly. Perform a crawling motion from your hands and feet by moving opposite limbs forward at the same time. When transitioning from side to side, do not rush. Make sure that your hips stay low with your knees close to the ground and that your core is tight with your back flat to slightly arched upward. When you have mastered the slow bear crawl pattern, work in a variation with a faster pace and for longer duration. You can also work in backward crawls. These will bring out the kid in you!

Supine Progression:

"Supine" means to lie on your back facing upward. The exercises in this group are designed to focus on the front abdominals. The first position, the 90/90, is an excellent foundation of core stabilization. Perform three to five sets of thirty to sixty seconds or perform five to ten breaths per set. The other exercises are more repetition-based. For these, perform two to four sets of ten to fifteen repetitions per side, or three to five repetitions per side, holding the position for three to five breaths each time. Be careful not to overreach with your arms and legs at first. It is most important that you focus on the core, maintaining a neutral posture.

90/90 Holds (B)

Start on your back with your feet on a wall. The wall will help you get into the right position for this. Your hips and knees should be flexed to 90 degrees. Place your arms straight at your sides and lightly press them into the ground. You should notice that your core activates. Focus on tilting

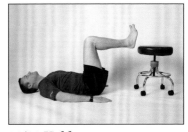

90/90 Holds.

your pelvis backward, lightly flattening your spine to the ground, and keeping your lower rib cage down. Pull your feet off the wall and hold this posture. If you are unable to hold this position, pull your knees a little more toward you. If it is too easy, you can drift your legs away slightly.

Leg Reach (I)

The next step is to add an alternating leg reach to the stable position. Assume the 90/90 position without the wall. Perform one leg reach

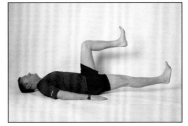

Leg Reach in supine.

straight out, touching your heel lightly to the ground, and then return to the starting position. Alternate reaches between legs. Pay close attention to your core control during this. Do not let your lower back arch or your lower ribs lift.

Alternating Arm and Leg Reach or "Dying Bug" (A)

Start in the same 90/90 position but with your arms also flexed at 90 degrees and pointing toward the ceiling. Perform alternating and opposite arm/leg reaches. Make sure to keep your core tight and hips and spine in place.

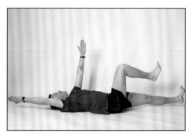

Dying bug.

Ball Pinch—Alternating Arm and Leg Reach (A)

To take the dying bug up one final notch, get your physio ball out. Place the ball between your knees and arms in the dying bug position. Press all four limbs into the ball, increasing your core activation. Now, perform the same dying bug as above by alternating opposite arms and legs.

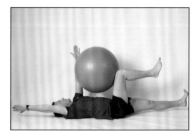

Alternating arm and leg reach with ball pinch.

The limbs that are not moving will be holding the ball. You will have to press diagonally to hold the ball. A larger ball will make this more challenging. Consider performing on one side at a time for a variation. For this, hold the ball between the same side arm and leg while the opposite side moves.

Half Kneel/Lunge Progression:

The half kneel and the lunge are important to master. These positions focus on stabilization of the core when your legs are in opposite positions, with one in front and one behind. This position mimics a running stride. It is key to this progression to maintain a neutral lumbar spine. If you are tighter through your iliopsoas and rectus femoris, the muscles in front of your hips and thighs, you may find this position hard to control. If this is the case, double back to the flexibility chapter before venturing into these exercises. The first position, the narrow half kneel hold, should be performed in two to four sets of thirty to sixty seconds a side, or perform five to ten breaths while holding a side. The other exercises are more repetition-based. For these, perform two to four sets of ten to fifteen repetitions per side.

Narrow Half-Kneel Hold (B)

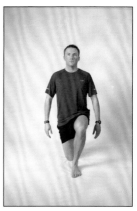

Perform a kneeling position with one knee down and the other in front. This should look like your iliopsoas stretch position. Perform a light tuck of your pelvis and hold. Now, move your foot in front and your knee/foot on the ground to as much of an inline posture as you can. Focus on controlling your torso in an erect posture.

Narrow half-kneel hold.

Chops (I)

Start in the kneeling position as above with your feet at shoulder width. You can narrow them later to further the challenge. Take a medicine ball or small dumbbell and hold this with both hands over your shoulder on the side that the knee is raised. Make a diagonal motion with your hands, like you are chopping wood, to the knee that is on the ground. Then reverse the motion and pull it back up to the high position. Make sure your trunk stays tall and your core is tight as you move the weight. After you have this pattern down, perform a faster arm movement, but still control it with a pause on the other end.

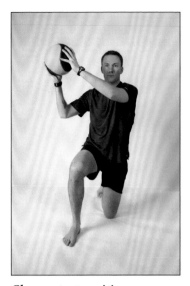

Chops, start position.

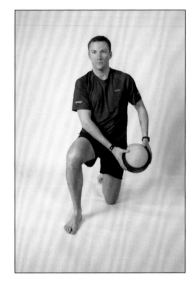

Chops, finish position.

Lunge Anti-Rotation Press (A)

Standing with one leg in front and one leg in back, lower your body down about six inches, and hold this position. Try to keep most of your weight on the lead leg. It is okay if you lean your torso slightly forward to do this. Hold a band in both hands with the other end attached to an object such as a

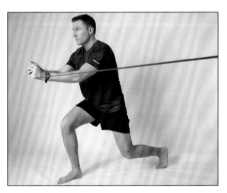

Lunge anti-rotation press.

door or a pole at chest height to your side. Now perform a bench press motion of the band by pressing both hands from your chest to straight in front of you. Make sure your core stays tight and does not move as you press out. Perform a set with each leg forward and pull the band each direction, left and right. Complete four sets in each position. Use a resistance band with more tension or try using a cable machine to challenge yourself more as it gets easier.

Knee Resisted Lunge (A)

This is a great variation of the lunge for a runner. Place a band around the outside of a knee and tie the other end to an object at the same height. Perform a standing lunge with the band trying to pull your knee inward. Do not let it. Keep your

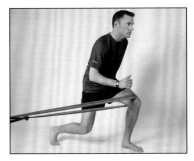

Knee resisted lunge.

foot and knee straight as well as your hips squared in the direction you are facing.

Lunge Ups (E)

Start in a half-knee position. Make sure your core is held tight. Follow a sequence: press your lead foot down by squeezing your glute on this side, shift your weight forward and lean with your torso, press down again with this leg, lifting the back knee about one inch off the ground, hold this position

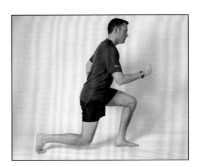

Lunge ups.

for three to five seconds, then return to the starting position. Each step should be performed slowly with each rep. It's harder than it seems.

Standing Progression:

The final stabilization group focuses on standing positions. This is where you function from as a runner, so it is essential that you can control your body here. Perform two to four sets on each side for the first three, or each direction for the helicopter.

Resisted Arm Swing (B)

Stand on one leg with your knee slightly bent. Shift your weight forward on the foot that is on the ground. Make sure not to bend forward from your hips; instead, position your core in neutral and hold it tight. Now perform an alternating arm swing with a dumbbell in each hand, like you are running. Allow your forearms to lightly brush your sides and with your hands landing close to your belly button. Make sure to keep your foot, knee, hips, and shoulder pointing in the direction you are facing. If you are able to do this, swing your arms with more force and try using heavier weights.

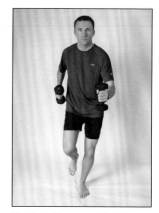

Resisted arm swing balance.

Resisted Knee Raises (I)

Stand on one leg in the same posture as above. Place a band around the outside of the opposite knee with the other end tied at mid-thigh level. The band should run in front of the leg that is on the ground and attach to the other leg that is farther from the band. Perform slow knee raises, making sure to control your leg in a straight plane while you keep your torso and foot/knee on the ground straight. Increase the resistance as tolerated.

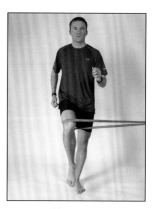

Resisted knee raises.

Suitcase Carry (I)

The suitcase carry has the same purpose as the suitcase squat but applies movement. Hold a weight with one hand at your side. Stand tall, making sure your torso does not lean one way or the other. Keep your core

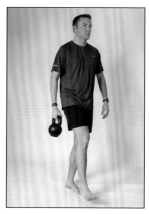

Suitcase carry.

engaged and neutral. Now, slowly walk forward. If you are able to control the weight well, try more resistance. Perform this on each side.

Helicopters (E)

This is a fun exercise, but takes more space to perform safely and requires some equipment. Use a thicker rope with light resistance firmly tied to the end. A four-foot section of rope with a soft ankle weight works well. Stand in squat position but only part of the way

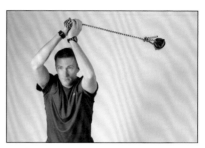

Helicopters.

down, and perform a circular motion with your hands and arm, spinning the weight with the rope overhead. Focus on pulsing through your core at one point in each revolution. Do not just spin the rope through your arms and shoulders. Vary the point of pulse such as in front of you, to the side, or the back. Then switch directions.

Quality and Quantity of Core Stabilization

This completes the exercises to fine-tune your core strength and stabilization. Remember, quality is more important than quantity. Getting through twenty repetitions of higher resistance with bad form is never going to be as beneficial as doing a few well-controlled repetitions. Also, always focus on posture and breath control. Consider performing these exercises in front of a mirror, so that you can see what you're doing. If you do not have a mirror available, consider having a friend watch you or film you.

When setting up a core program, variety is important. At a minimum, runners should do a core session two or three days a week. I recommend picking two or three exercises from each of the categories in this chapter. Vary your selection each day by picking from different groups or progressions. One thing to consider is the position that the exercise is performed in—pick one each that is on your back, side, kneeling, and then standing, instead of exercises that are all done in the same position. They will all activate your core differently. If you follow this plan, you will perform four to six exercises each day, which should take only fifteen to twenty minutes. In total, that means thirty to sixty minutes per week. This is well worth the small amount of time to decrease your risk of injury and help your running economy and performance. For more guidance on structuring your core program, see the appendix.

As important as all of these exercises are, we need to put this strength and stability to use. In the next chapter you will learn how to use the strength and stability you're building to power your running engine.

Chapter 9

Running Mechanics Reeducation

Spend some time mastering the exercises from the previous two chapters. This will help you to build a solid foundation for your core. However, even when you have all of this strength in the foundation, you still need to apply it to your running. It's kind of like buying a brand new, finely tuned car. The engine may have a lot of power and run smoothly, but if you do not balance and align the tires on the car, the engine is useless. When you drive, the car will just wobble and veer all over the road.

Think about the last time you were running behind someone and watching his mechanics. You watch his arms flail side to side, torso twisting, and a funky whip kick thing making his legs look like a windmill. It is amazing this runner isn't injured. Maybe some clamshell exercises would help strengthen his glutes and help with leg control. Or perhaps some planks would stiffen his core. Unfortunately, he could strengthen his hips and stabilize his core for weeks, but he wouldn't run any differently. Mechanics are rooted much deeper. Changing running form requires retraining, not just strengthening.

When you learn a new task, it takes concentration to put the components together. After a number of repetitions, the pieces start to flow more easily. You do not need to think as much and they just kind of happen at an unconscious level. This is essential for running.

Recall from our discussion of gait mechanics in Chapter 2 that the average gait cycle takes a half to three-quarters of a second. This does not allow a lot of time to think, especially when one stride is occurring immediately after the other, often around 150 to 200 times a minute. The rapid pace and number of repetitions make application of your core stabilization crucial. To do this, it takes practice—and a lot of it. Depending on how many aspects of your form you're trying to change, it will likely take months of dedication to engrain the tweaks. Then, as with your car, you'll need to do some routine maintenance along the way to keep things running smoothly.

Before diving into running-specific drills, it is important to apply your core stability to more dynamic activities. The following drills will bridge the gap from the previously learned static stabilization to more movement-based control.

This is the time to put it all together. Review the video you took of yourself in Chapter 5. What were the quirks that jumped out at you? Focus on these areas, your body posture, and control of your core. It is a lot to think about, which is why it will take some time to make changes. Start slowly, focusing on one thing at a time and adding others as you go. Use a mirror for feedback. This visualization will provide immediate feedback, helping to hone in on the correct posture. Finally, have someone take video of you every few weeks. This will give you more feedback to make sure it is all coming together as it should.

The more you do these drills, the easier and more refined they will become. At a minimum, perform them on half of your run days each week. They act as a good extension to the dynamic flexibility learned in Chapter 7. You can perform these drills before you start a run in anticipation of mimicking the movement patterns during the run. On days that you are running faster or performing speed work, do them as part of your warm-up. I am also an advocate for more drills after your run. Many people lose their form when they fatigue, making post-run drills even more important for efficiency and injury reduction. If you can control your core and posture after a hard run, you are in good shape.

If appropriate, take your shoes off for these drills. This will help strengthen your feet and legs and allow you to better feel your body's position and contact on the ground. It will also improve ground-to-body and body-to-brain reaction times, helping to speed the subconscious training. Try to do at least 50 percent of your drills per week without shoes. Occasionally using your shoes will help to connect the dots to your running. Now, let's balance the wheels on your car and get you running.

To Start: Get Your Body in the Right Position

Posture is essential to efficient running form. Take what you have learned in Chapters 6 and 8 and apply it here. Your body should be straight through your ankles, hips, shoulders, and ears. Be cautious as you stand tall that you do not overextend your lower back. Maintain a neutral tuck of the pelvis and don't allow your lower back to arch excessively forward. Tracing this up the chain, the lower rib cage should remain down and your eyes facing forward. Keep your shoulders relaxed downward and slightly retracted backward, opening up your chest. Now, allow your weight to shift slightly forward on your feet. Pretend you're doing a plank in the air by maintaining a tight core and a straight body—your shift has to occur at your ankles. Your heels should remain on the ground. This forward shift brings your body into a position that is better for running.

The Segway gets its name from the two-wheeled, self-balancing personal transportation machine. Segways move forward and back when the rider shifts her weight in the direction she wants to go. If you lean forward, the wheels move faster to get underneath you and prevent you from falling. It's the same in running. The Segway drill acts as a gas pedal. Shift your weight a little forward, you start to jog. Shift a little more, and you run. The key is maintaining your straight posture. The degree of lean for distance runners will be small. The following drills are important to master, but can be incorporated into times when you're just standing, rather than only pre- or post-run.

Two-Leg Segway

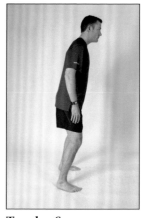

Stand with your feet shoulder-width apart. Make sure your feet and knees point straight ahead. Splay your toes open and press the pads of the toes into the ground. Bend your knees about 30 degrees. Focusing on neutral hip and spine posture, shift your weight forward to the front of your feet but keep your heels on the ground. You should feel about 60-75 percent of your weight in the front portion of your feet. Perform three repeti-

Two-leg Segway.

tions, holding for sixty seconds each interval. This is an easy but important drill. After you have mastered this exercise, incorporate it throughout the day. The carryover to running will be even better.

One-Leg Segway "Midstance"

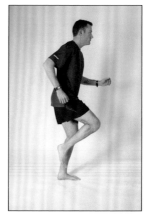

To make your posture more running-specific, take the two-leg Segway and perform it on one leg. Start in the two-leg Segway position, then shift your weight to one side. Lift the other leg up with your knee bent in front and your ankle underneath your body. Control your posture and keep your hips level, left to right. Keep your weight forward on your foot, and, finally, make sure your knee does not cave inward.

One-leg Segway "Midstance."

A light flex of your outer hip and glutes will help with this. If needed, hold on to a wall or chair to help balance.

Perform three repetitions of thirty to sixty seconds on each leg. Increase the length of the hold as it becomes easier. Again, this is a great exercise to perform during the day. Maybe it is harder to perform this at the office, but you could always do it while brushing your teeth.

Now Swing Your Arms

The way you swing your arms is a reflection of what the rest of your body is doing. By working on core control and leg alignment, your arms will likely naturally swing in the right position. And by improving arm swing control, the rest of your body will follow. Think of your opposite arm and leg as counterbalancing each other. This is a progression of drills, working from a sitting position to kneeling, lunging, and then standing posture. If you are new to mechanics drills, start in the sitting position and work your way up. After you have worked your way through these, focus on the standing position. Similar to the Segway drills, you won't need to revisit these exercises after you've mastered control. They will be incorporated with many of the other drills.

Core Controlled Arm Swing Progression

Sit on the ground with your legs straight out in front of you. Make sure your torso is vertical. If not, bend your knees slightly and review the earlier flexibility and mobility information to loosen the area. Now keep your core tight and swing your arms like you are running. Keep the tops of your shoulders and neck relaxed, opening your chest by slightly drawing your shoulders

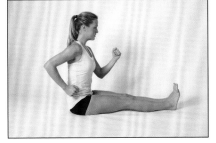

Core-controlled arm swing, long sit posture.

backward. Depress your elbows slightly away from your shoulders. Your elbows should stay bent at 90 degrees. Your swing point should occur at the shoulder. Allow your hands to swing toward midline in front of you, but stop before they cross the belly button. Make sure your hands are relaxed. I like to think of holding a potato chip between my thumb and index finger while keeping a loose fist. As you swing forward and back, your forearms should lightly brush your sides. When the arm is behind you, your hand should land at your hip. Start slowly and increase the speed as you improve. Start with three repetitions of one minute. When this is well-controlled and easy to perform, work your way through the following postures: long sit with feet in front, half kneeling like you are doing the half-kneel stability hold, the upright position of a lunge, and the resisted arm swing exercise as outlined in Chapter 8.

Begin Applying the Movement

The following five drills focus on core and movement control. They increase warmth and activation patterns pre-running. Concentrate on staying light on your feet during all of these. Pretend that you are landing on hot coals and do not want to burn your feet. The pace at which these next five drills should be performed is quick but not forced. Your movement should feel smooth and controlled. Perform two or three laps of a fifty-foot distance if you have a long enough space available. If not, perform three to five laps of a twenty-five-foot distance.

Butt Kicks

Butt kicks exaggerate activation of the hamstring and drawing your foot off of the ground. Keeping your core tight, control your arm swing by alternating kicks back with your feet, trying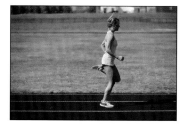

Butt Kicks.

to kick your butt with your heel. Allow your legs to be relaxed. The movement should not feel forced.

High Knees

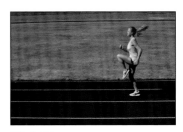

High Knees.

High knees isolate iliopsoas activation and lifting your leg off the ground. Focus on snapping your leg off the ground and lifting your knee up in front of you. Keep the front foot flexed as you raise your knee. Only go as high as you can while still maintaining core and trunk control. If you are forced to lean backward, decrease the height that you are lifting your knee. Make sure to incorporate arm swing here as well.

Shuffle

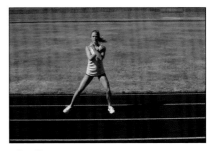

Shuffle.

The sideways shuffle will wake up the outer glutes and hip muscula-ture. Perform a slight squat with your knees bent to 30 degrees. Shuffle sideways, maintaining an engaged core with feet and knees pointing straight ahead. Keep a small gap between your feet when you bring your legs together with each stride. Perform an arm swing motion during this, like you are doing jumping jacks. When your feet are apart, your arms should be overhead, and when your legs are together, your hands should be together at midline by your abdomen.

Karaoke

The karaoke or grapevine will also work on the lateral stabiliz-ers of the core. This incorporates an important rotational stability necessary for the running stride. Stand tall and, as always, keep your core tight. Perform an alternating crossover of your feet by first stepping in front and then behind the opposite leg. As you cross over in front with the lead leg, exaggerate your knee raise

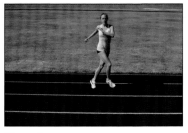

Karaoke.

slightly. Swing your arms like you are running but allow them to rotate with your torso as you go. Make sure you are light on your feet.

Skater Hops

The skater hop is a diagonal bounding drill that focuses on recruitment of the lateral core stabilizers while placing heavy emphasis on lower-extremity alignment. Start in the one-leg Segway position, like you are in midstance of your running stride. Perform a diagonal forward hop, landing on the opposite side in the same midstance position. Make sure that you are soft in your landing, allowing your knee to bend when you contact the ground. Make sure your core is tight and your foot and knee are

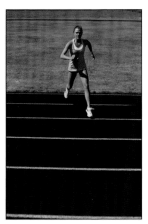

Skater hops.

pointed in the direction you want to go. As long as you are able to land with good control, you can perform this in a more plyometric fashion, at a faster pace. Just make sure that you do not sacrifice speed for control.

Lift Your Feet Off the Ground

Now that your body is falling into alignment and moving freely, focus on your hip drive. As you leave the stance phase of gait and transition into swing, it is important to focus on lifting your leg from the ground with your hip flexors. This will improve your overall turnover. As you think of this concept during these drills, envision running on sand or ice. If you push off hard in sand or ice, your foot will slip backward, causing you to lose power. Instead, draw the leg up quickly through your hip to get your leg forward and keep your stride rolling. As a runner, you want to spend your energy moving forward, not up and down. Focusing on hip drive will help you to minimize vertical displacement.

Wall Drill

Place both hands on a wall like you were doing a plank from a standing push-up position. Make sure your body is angled forward. Start with one knee raised and bent upward, and rise up on your toes on the down leg. Now lower your lead leg to the ground and lift your opposite leg about one inch, then quickly snap your lead leg back up and pause. The focus should be on

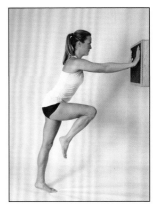

Wall Drill.

the rise of your lead leg back to the starting position. Perform three sets of ten repetitions with each leg.

Marching A

After mastering the wall drill, progress toward a forward moving march. The mechanics are the same but arm swing is incorporated. Instead of focusing on one leg at a time, it will be performed in an alternating fash-

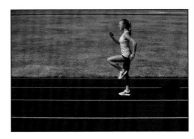

Marching A.

ion. Make sure the change of your feet from side to side is quick, but well controlled through your core. Follow the same parameters for the drills earlier, performing two or three laps of fifty feet or three to five laps of twenty-five feet.

100-Ups

This is a drill that focuses on endurance and control. It is similar to the wall drill, but without hand support and more of a simultaneous motion. This drill is performed in place without moving forward. Stand on one leg in your one-leg Segway position. Quickly lift the leg from the ground, raising your knee upward while your other leg falls back to the ground. Pause briefly and then continue with an alternating motion between the legs. The goal is to complete one set of fifty repetitions on each side while maintaining good body control.

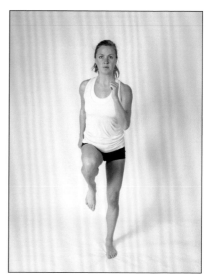

100-Ups.

Then Control Your Leg Movement in the Air

Many of the drills up to this point have focused on getting the leg off the ground and controlling it while it is in stance. It is important that we emphasize how to get the leg back to the ground. We want to pull the foot backward as it makes contact with the ground. We do not want your leg to be swinging forward when it contacts initially. To do this, think about pawing back.

Scuffing "Charging Bulls"

Stand in your midstance position on one leg. The leg that is in the air will be your focus leg for the drill. Pretend you have gum on the ball of your foot and you are trying to scuff it off. Perform a quick circular motion from the up position, brushing your foot briefly on the ground as it goes underneath you. The contact

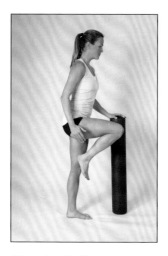

Charging bulls start.

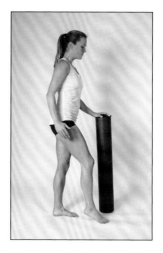

Charging bulls at scuff point on ground.

point should be just in front of your toes but to the side from your foot on the ground. Pause when it returns to the high position. Focus on a quick snapping motion. You may need to hold on to something when you first begin this drill. Perform three sets of ten to fifteen repetitions with each leg. Progress to hands-free as able and perform a running arm swing motion with the scuff.

Marching B

The Marching B is similar to the A but focuses more on controlling the leg as it moves in front of you. It places more focus on hamstring activation. Perform a Marching A, but when your knee is up, reach your foot out in front like you are

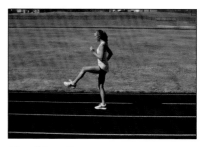

Marching B.

taking a stride, and then pull it back underneath as you did with the charging bulls. Just as you did with the Marching A, aim for two or three laps of fifty feet or three to five laps of twenty-five feet.

Control Your Body at Impact

Band Running

Place a long resistance band around your waist and anchor it to a sturdy object such as a high table leg or a tree, at the same level behind you. Move forward to create tension on the band so that you are forced to lean forward slightly into the resistance. Now, march in place. If you are able to control the march well, run in place. Make sure your core is

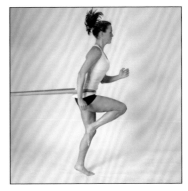

Band running.

tight and you are not hinging forward at your waist. Remember to lead with your hips over your toes. This is best performed in timed intervals—aim for three repetitions of one minute each.

Runner Hop

Think of the runner hop as a slow-motion run. This is one of the best tests to see if you have all of the pieces of the running puzzle ready to go. Alternate a one-foot hop forward as if you are running. Your feet should almost follow a line that is on the ground, maybe just a little wider. Land lightly on a flatter foot, not your heel, with your knee slightly bent. Pay close attention to your foot, knee, and hip alignment. Do two or three laps of fifty feet or three to five laps of twenty-five feet.

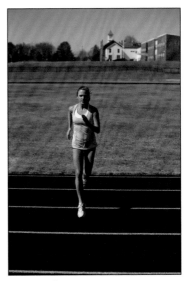

Runner hop.

Land Softly by Disbursing the Load Through Your Body Like a Spring

Landing softly is important because if you are lighter on your feet, then your impact is disbursed more evenly throughout the joints and muscles. This is important to decrease stress on your joints. To improve running economy, land softly and teach your muscles to act like springs, which is what they are designed to do. Runners who have a faster stride turnover spend less time with their feet on the ground, which creates less stress on the body. Their feet will be less "sticky" and appear free-flowing as they quickly land and spring from the ground. Improve turnover by tracking cadence. This can be done using a simple hand-held metronome. If you are not musically inclined, download a metronome app and target 180 beats per minute or more for the following drills. This number is selected because it mimics the fast rate at which our muscles rebound when loaded.

Cadence Hopping

Start with a two-foot hop in place with a cadence of 180 beats per minute. Focus on landing light and soft on the ground. You should land first on your toes but allow your heels to lightly kiss the ground with each repetition. After you can match the cadence, perform on one leg at a time. The height of your hop will be dictated more by the cadence at which you are jumping. Start with three repetitions of one minute. For variety, try jumping rope to the cadence.

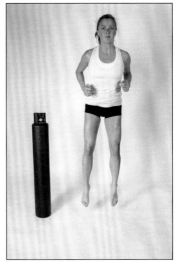

Cadence hopping.

Running in Place

Running in place is an excellent way to start putting all the pieces together. Focus on core control, arm swing, lifting your feet underneath you off the ground, and being light on your feet. You can perform this to cadence as well. You may need to start slower than 180 steps per minute and work your way up. It is also fine to perform cadences that are higher than 180, which may be required for speed work or faster-paced running. If you have heard of the ankling drill, running in place is similar to this but more specific to running because it focuses more on the knee leg lift. To combine the two, perform the run in place in a slow-moving forward fashion as well. I know this is not running in place, but it still has the same concept. Perform three repetitions of one minute.

Skipping A

If you have not skipped in a while, you need to. It is a great way to rekindle some of the movement patterns of your youth while encouraging better running mechanics. Start with a basic school-yard skip. You will notice that you land more on the

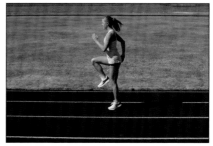

Skipping A.

mid or front portion of the foot. Now, increase the speed at which you turn your feet and arms over. Do not lose control of your core as you pick up the pace, and stay light on your feet. Perform two or three laps of a fifty-foot distance if you have a long enough space available; if not, perform three to five laps of a twenty-five-foot distance.

Skipping B

The next step is to add the reach and paw-back motion. This should look the same as it did with your Marching B and the charging bull exercises. To get going, perform your Skipping A, then add the forward reach and pull back as you go. Again, perform two or three laps of fifty feet or three to five laps of twenty-five feet.

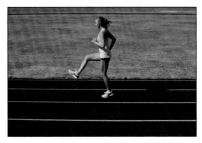

Skipping B.

Bounding

Think of bounding as a plyometric run, meaning that your stride is going to open up and have more of a hop to it. Spring from one foot to the other. Allow your body to land softly but then quickly explode back up. It is okay to have a little more up-and-down motion than

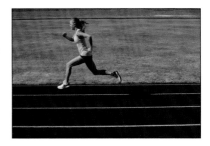

Bounding.

you normally do when you run. Each time you transition from one side to the other, quickly drive your knee up while driving your opposite arm forward. Do two or three laps of fifty feet or three to five laps of twenty-five feet.

Perform This Over and Over While You Run

Now that you have practiced all of the components, you need to start running. These are two drills that make this transition easier.

Fall into Running and Striders

Run in place first, focusing on the key mechanics of running. Slowly apply the Segway falling motion, allowing your body to run forward. Keep your core tight while you run a brief distance. Turn around, reset by running in place, and return.

This completes a solid group of running drills. You do not need to perform all of these every time you do your drill work. Home in more on the drills that focus on the areas where you have weaknesses. The more you can fine-tune your running mechanics, the more efficient your stride will become. Along with this comes easier, smoother, faster, and less injury-prone running. As I have heard before and personally keep in the back of my mind with my training, improvement in running form is free speed. Spend some time with these, even if it means sacrificing some running time, and they will repay you in the long run.

The past four chapters stressed the importance of figuring out and improving your foundation of running. This is important, even though it may not be as fun as running itself. However, if you look at the hours in your week, the time spent doing these exercises and drills, and even your running, is really only a drop in the bucket. There are a number of other hours that we can't forget about as they may be just as, if not more, important to our overall running core health. In the final chapter we will look at posture and activities of daily living that have a direct impact on our running core health.

Chapter 10

Core Health for When You're Not Running

You wake up in the morning and start to think about running. Should you head out the door before the day gets going, wait until your lunch break, or try to squeeze it in before dinner? Where will you go? Maybe some local trails, the roads, or a treadmill at the gym? How far should you run and at what pace? After reading about your core, I hope there is more to this thought process. You need to make sure your core is fit to run. Core health is an expression of not only mobility, flexibility, stability, and strength but also footwear, daily posture, occupation, sleep, diet, and most other things that happen in the many hours a day you are not running.

As a health care professional who works daily with orthopedic injuries, I will be the first to say that the majority of runners' injuries are not just orthopedic. It is easy to think that "runner's knee" is just a pain in the knee that will improve with rest, ice, stretching, and strengthening, but think deeper than this. Consider other variables that have a direct relationship to running, such as footwear, running surface and terrain, and training parameters such as intensity and volume. Everyday decisions can also influence your running, like footwear, sleeping position, driving posture, diet, stress, and your posture during the day at work and home. Even if you run seven days a week for sixty to ninety minutes each day, that only makes up about

5 percent of your total week. Be mindful of the other 95 percent that can affect your core health just as much—if not more than—your running.

Footwear

How much time did you put into buying your running shoes? Most runners read about running shoes, speak with their running friends about them, and then have someone watch the way they walk and run at a running shop before making the purchase. Footwear is a popular topic in most running crowds because when you look at running attire, this is the one piece that affects your running the most. Do you wear a thin, barebones pair of minimalist shoes? Or how about a big, thick, high-rise pair of maximalist shoes? What about all of the more traditional running shoes?

Now, what about daily lifestyle footwear, the ones you might wear for dozens of hours per week? Most people hop online and order a pair, hoping they come in the right size, or maybe walk into a shop, try them on, and take them home. You probably put more thought into the fashion of your street shoes than the function.

Let me paint a picture for you. I am at work in an active ortho-pedic sports physical clinic. People are jumping, running, and doing exercises all around me. An injured businesswoman, who is a runner, comes in on her lunch break complaining of plantar fasciitis. She sits down and explains how her plantar fasciitis will not go away and has been bothering her for months. She has changed running shoes three times since it has started, tried some stretch-ing, but nothing seems to help. The first question she asks is, "What running shoes should I be wearing?" Then, I look at her feet and see three-inch heels.

This three-inch heel is the shoe that the patient wears ten hours a day. If this patient with plantar fasciitis has tightness of her calf, she could stretch for an hour a day and likely not see improvement. Every time she puts the heels back on, the calf is shortened, which trickles up the chain, shortening the hamstring, shutting off the glutes, and driving the pelvis more forward, out of the neutral position that you have been aiming for all along. So for ten hours a day, her core is in the wrong position, not setting her up for a good run that afternoon.

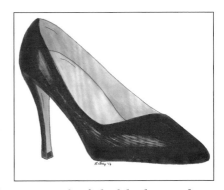

An example of a high heel-to-toe drop.

Now, think about stiff, rigid work boots. Someone wearing them day in and day out is restricting the natural movement of the foot. Look at the arch in your foot. This is designed to be a spring, flattening a bit as your foot loads onto the ground, then returning the energy with a rebound as it leaves the ground. If you wrap your foot in a hard leather and rubber boot, the natural spring will not work effectively. If shock absorption is decreased, an increased load will be placed on the joints of the legs and spine.

Also, the thicker and harder-soled shoe minimizes the amount of feedback that the body gets from the ground. Consider a hot stove. If you touched one, the receptors in your hand would trigger a quick reaction to pull your hand away, hopefully before it was burned. Now, if you had a thin glove on your hand and touched the same stove, the heat would take a second before triggering the same reaction. In heavy oven mitts, you might not feel the heat at all. The same goes for your foot. The more you place between the foot and the ground, the less sensation you will receive and at a delayed pace. We need fast and appropriate timing of our muscles. If the foot is delayed, the other structures through the core will be as well. This does not mean you need to go barefoot, but if you are in a leather boot all day, a transition to a running shoe may be abrupt for your body.

Finally, visualize a men's dress shoe. Think about how the front is narrow and maybe even has a pointy toe box. Does a foot look the

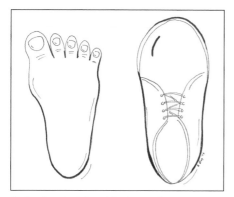

Baby foot with wide toe splay.
Rounded toe box shoe can
accommodate this foot well.

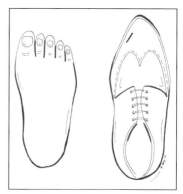

Adult foot with crammed
toes and bunion formation.
The foot needs to look like
this to fit into a dress shoe.

same? Well, maybe think of a baby's foot, which is narrow through the heel and wide in the toe box, with a nice splay of the toes. The foot is designed to allow the toes to grab the ground during movement. These are the anchors of the body and essential to overall stability. If we place that tiny foot in a hard dress shoe with a narrower toe box, the foot would not be able to splay naturally. This confined toe box would limit the ability of the toes to activate and move properly. Without proper movement, the plantar fascia does not function appropriately and the rest of the movement cascade is negatively affected.

So, what should you look for in your non-running shoes?

Heel-to-Toe Drop

Heel-to-toe drop is the difference in height from the back of the shoe to the front of the shoe. A shoe that is more level in these measurements, thus having a lower heel, is ideal.

Flexible

The shoe's sole should be able to bend to allow, not hinder, movement of the foot.

Thin

A thinner sole will allow better feedback from the ground to your body.

Toe Box Width

A wider toe box will allow the front of the foot and toes to splay naturally, helping to improve movement patterns.

The running shoe, although quite important, is not the only piece of the footwear discussion. Lifestyle shoes need to be strongly considered to help runners improve their core health and overall running. Of course, there are certain times that the function or style of the shoe is necessary for safety or fashion. I am not saying that you can never wear that higher heel or work boot, but be mindful of the amount of time that you spend in them. Also, if you decide to make a footwear change, do it slowly. Our bodies adapt over time. If you have been wearing a shoe for months or even years, the transition to something different may take months or even years. Introduce the new shoe gradually while listening to your body to make sure an injury is not brewing.

Sitting

You may have heard that sitting is the new smoking. What does this mean? Basically, sitting is not good for you. Think back to Chapter 6 when we talked about the neutral core and proper standing posture. Sitting is not good posture—it's not natural. The more you sit, the more you hinder your running.

Most people are required to sit most of the day at work, which influences the angles of your joints and your hip and spine posture.

When you're sitting in a chair, your hips are flexed about 90 degrees, knees bent to 90 degrees, and your arms are in front, most likely on a keyboard. Now picture your running posture. The two scenarios have few similarities in the angles of your joints. One of the primary negative factors is the hip angle.

By placing your hip at 90 degrees and holding it for long durations, your iliopsoas is in a shortened position. The longer you remain seated, the more your body adapts to this position. When you stand up to walk, something has to give. If your hip flexor is tight, either your torso will be bent forward from the hip when you walk or your torso will be vertical, but your hips will be tilted forward with your lumbar spine rounded forward. This sets someone up for the open scissors posture. You could try to correct it by stretching the hip flexor and stabilizing the core in neutral, but if we do not change or limit sitting during the day, it is going to be an uphill battle. Sitting for eight hours a day and stretching for a few minutes are never going to balance each other out.

The first change is to minimize the amount of time you sit. Limit static sitting to no more than twenty minutes at a time. Use a timer at your desk to cue a position change. When the timer goes off, get up and move. Go to the bathroom, get a drink, do five squats, anything to break the sitting monotony. If it is not realistic to leave your sitting area, change position at minimum. Try kneeling on one knee as though you were doing a hip flexor stretch. You can vary this knee from side to side. Maybe kneel on both knees. Stand for a while. As you are standing, try to vary your position as well. Shift from one leg to the other, place one foot in front on a small step or chair, or try holding a small bend in your knees. The key to all of this is variety. Humans are not meant to be stationary, so the more movement you can build into the day, the better.

If you are stuck sitting, do it with better posture. Slouching at your desk or on the couch rounds your lower back, increasing the load on your spine. This causes your shoulders to slouch and your head likely to protrude forward. You would not want to run in this posture, so try not to sit like this either.

Think of a straight spine, which does not need to be vertical. If you are working on a laptop computer or work on top of your desk, leaning forward may be better. To do this, sit toward the front of

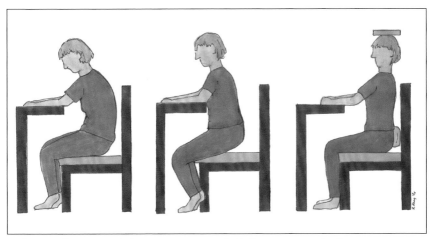

Left to right: Poor sitting posture; good sitting posture for laptop or top-of-desk work; good sitting posture for work using a computer monitor.

your chair, not using the back support. Bend your feet underneath you slightly so that your knees are closer to the floor than your hips. If you are using a monitor that is positioned at eye level, your spine will be better positioned if it is closer to vertical. To help with this, try holding a book on top of your head. If it stays in position, you are probably not tipping your head too far downward. But, again, try a variety of positions.

If you have to remain sitting, vary the position above by occasionally using the back rest. Placing a small rolled towel behind your lower back will help to cue a better core position. Another variation is shifting your weight from right to left by increasing the amount of pressure in one sit bone over the other. You can also rotate your hips, dropping one farther back in the seat than the other. Just remember to move—it may not be walking or standing, but it at least creates variety.

Recall the No Money exercise in Chapter 6. This is a great exercise to perform throughout the day. It is not designed to fatigue you, but rather to wake up and cue better posture. Keep a light resistance band near your workstation and try performing fifteen repetitions every hour or two during the day. This should help you remain active.

Driving

Cars are made for comfort, which is not always best for your core. If you drive less than twenty minutes a day, I would not be concerned. But, if you spend much of your day in and out of the car, you need to rethink driving posture.

With most cars you will likely be slightly reclined in your seat, and that is okay. Make sure the seat is not tipped back too far. Also pay attention to the bottom of the seat that you sit on. It should be relatively flat so that your hips are close to—or just above—the height of your knees, which can be hard to do with some seats. Sitting with a small towel rolled under your hips or on top of a wedge cushion will help to optimally align your core. A built-in lumbar support or rolled-up towel behind your lower back can also help to remind you of better posture. It should not force a new position, but remind you to maintain it.

A cue that I use when I am driving longer distances is to pay attention to what I see in my mirrors. Look at them when you first get in your car. If they are positioned well, you should be able to see the desired spaces around you. As you drive, the tendency is to slouch more, making it harder to see out of your mirrors, especially the rear-view. Don't adjust your mirror when this happens. Instead, sit back up and make sure you can see out of the mirrors as you could when you started. This will help to keep you in a better posture.

Standing

We looked at standing posture at length in Chapter 6. Keep the neutral core position in mind especially. Do not allow yourself to over-relax by letting your breathing and core position go. If you are standing for longer periods of time, make small changes to your position as much as possible. Shift your weight side to side or place one knee on a low step or stool in front of you. You can also use the Segway drill from Chapter 9 to help with standing posture. By incorporating one minute of this every so often while standing, it will help to keep your core active. Using a standing workstation can also be beneficial.

Walking

As you transition from standing to walking, remember the neutral pelvis and spine. Use a relaxed arm swing that should be even from side to side. Keep your head up with your eyes looking out in front of you. If you are walking for a longer distance, try rotating your palms so that they are facing forward. Hold this position for a few arm swings. This will help open your chest and shoulders.

Sleeping

Sleeping is non–weight bearing and will not affect your core much. However, it can't be forgotten because it makes up a good chunk of your time. Sleeping on your back or side tends to lend itself to better alignment. If you are a back sleeper, lie down on your back on a firm surface. If this is uncomfortable or your back arches high off the mattress, try sleeping with a small pillow under your knees at night. If you are sleeping on your side, bend your knees slightly but not too much. The more bent they are, the more your hip will be in a shortened position. Place a small pillow between your knees so that your hips and spine are straighter while you sleep.

Daily Movement

It is important to recognize how your daily movements aside from walking can negatively or positively affect your core and running. We are going to focus on two movements: a squat and a forward bend.

The squat is important for life. It is a movement pattern that humans start at around twelve to eighteen months of age. We squat to sit and stand from a chair, car, and in the bathroom. Squatting should also be used to lift an object, especially if it is heavier, from the ground. As often as we do this, we need to do it well. Refer back to good squat mechanics in Chapter 8. Integrate these as much as possible during the day. It will reinforce better movement patterns and decrease the stress on your joints.

Bending is just as important as squatting. When you're not able to squat and need to forward bend instead, focus on hinging from your hips and less on bending from your spine. A hip-hinge pattern for bending will replicate the Romanian dead lift covered in Chapter 8. Similar to the squat, focus on this movement during your daily activities.

Nutrition

I am not a nutrition expert and will not go in depth here. However, nutrition is essential to core health and healthy living, so it can't go unmentioned.

Someone who is overweight with more stored fat in the abdominal and gluteal region will be challenged to achieve a healthy core position. Picture someone who has a large stomach. This distends the abdominal wall and core musculature. If this area is overly stretched, it will not be able to function well, limiting the ability to hold a neutral core position. Without this position, optimal running mechanics will be difficult.

My recommendations on nutrition:

Educate yourself.
Don't just listen to one source of information. There is a lot of good but also poor literature circulating today. You need to be educated to make the best selection for yourself and your needs. Try searching the following for credible information: Nutrition.gov, U.S. National Library of Medicine, American Society for Nutrition, or the Nutrition Source offered by Harvard School of Public Health.

Ask for help.

Speak with an expert on nutrition to review your personal nutrition and help guide you in a direction that is best for you. Anyone can call him- or herself a nutritionist; this does not represent certification or licensure. Look for someone who is a Registered Dietitian Nutritionist or Certified Nutrition Specialist. These individuals have gone through a degree program, passed an exam, and a hold a license to practice nutrition.

Balance calories in and calories out.

Nutrition in a basic way can be viewed as a balance between the calories that you consume through eating compared to the calories that you expend through basic human function, such as breathing, thinking, and exercise. If you take in more calories than you expend, the extra calories need to be stored in your body and your weight will go up. In contrast, if you expend more calories than you consume, your weight will go down.

Quality over quantity.

I like to think of the quality of a calorie as the type of wood you put in a wood stove. If you put a piece of hardwood in a stove, it will take a while to burn. However, if you put a piece of soft wood in the same fire, it will burn much faster. Similarly, if you burn fat or protein, it will take longer, meaning that your energy will last longer into a run. If you burn granules of sugar, they will disappear much faster, causing you to fatigue or creating a need to replace them as you go.

Less packaging is usually better.

The more layers of boxes, wrappers, and sealants that are on something usually translates to more processing. Look for whole, natural foods or those that are less processed.

Fewer ingredients are preferable.

Compare two tomato sauces. One has three ingredients and the other has fifteen. The one with three ingredients likely has what it needs and less of what it does not need. The one that has numerous ingredients likely has high fructose corn syrup, fillers, and preservatives that are not necessary and unhealthy. Avoid foods that are genetically modified, pesticide-sprayed, contain growth hormone, or come from an antibiotic-fed source.

You are what you eat.

Eating healthy is critical to staying healthy. If you eat junk, you will have a poor foundation for your general health.

This covers many of the things that we do day in and day out that affect our core. If you do a good job of the basics, it sets you up for less maintenance overall, which means more time for the fun stuff, like running. The exercises and drills that we covered in Chapters 6 through 9 are easier to perform with better focus on daily core health. The more you integrate your health with your lifestyle, the less injury-prone and more efficient you will become.

Now, take what you have learned in this book and make your core healthier. It's for your own good. Just remember: Variety is a key to life; listen to your body—it will tell you if something is not right; and smile when you run. Running is an amazing gift, so savor the time when you are turning the legs over.

Keep on running.

Appendix:
Structuring a Core Routine

You now have all of the pieces to put together a complete core routine. Thinking back on everything you have learned may seem a little overwhelming or even unrealistic to schedule into your training. The following should provide a foundation to structure your personal core conditioning program in a feasible manner. You can also work other areas of the body into this on the same days. For example, a strength exercise that you may be doing for your ankle could be added to your core stability and strength exercises that you are already performing.

Keep in mind that this is a framework rather than a one-size-fits-all schedule and that the pieces that lie within will vary from one individual to the next. Finally, depending on what your goals are with running, this routine may fluctuate during your training cycle. For example, you will likely decrease the amount of strengthening that you are doing for a few weeks before an important race. During this time, you may want to focus more on soft-tissue mobility and flexibility.

See the relevant chapters (referenced below) for how to perform the listed exercises.

Summary Core Routine

Breathing Exercises (Chapter 6)

Perform before core strength/stability exercises. Think of this as a warm-up to help encourage better body position during your workout. Spend three to five minutes if you are newer to these exercises. When they are well controlled, perform two to three minutes regularly before each routine. These can also be performed pre-running and pre-running drills as needed to help with posture and position. Pick two positions each time that you perform these and then vary this with each session.

Progression of Breathing Positions

1. On your back with feet supported, hips and knees at 90 degrees.
2. On your back with knees bent and feet flat on the ground.
3. On all fours, hands and knees.
4. On your back with legs flat.
5. Seated on low step with back slightly rounded.
6. Standing.

Soft-Tissue Mobility (Chapter 7)

Perform primarily on run days, plus on off days as needed.

Pre-Running: Thirty-second scan of each area most days of the week. Perform an extra thirty seconds on areas that are tighter.

Post-Running: Repeat on harder workout days, during periods of higher mileage, or when peaking for competition.

<u>Areas of Focus:</u>
- Adductors
- Hip Flexors
- Quadriceps
- TFL/IT Band
- Gluteus Medius and Outer Hip
- Gluteus Maximus
- Piriformis and Hip Rotators
- Hamstring
- Lower Back Soft Tissue
- Thoracic Spine

Static Stretching (Chapter 7)

Perform post-running and on non-running days. Incorporate pre-run as needed but after at least a ten-minute warm-up.

Perform two to three sets, holding each stretch for thirty to sixty seconds. Target the parts of your body that are tighter. You will likely not be doing all of these stretches each time.

- Adductors
- Iliopsoas
- Rectus Femoris/Iliopsoas
- TFL/ IT Band—Standing Banana
- Hamstring—Toe Touches
- Gluteus Maximus and Gluteus Medius
- Piriformis and Hip Rotators—Modified Pigeon
- Thoracic Spine Rotation
- Lumbar and Thoracic Spine—Child's Pose

Dynamic Stretching (Chapter 7)

Perform on runs days, pre-running, and during a run as needed.

The Big Eight for Twenty-Five

Perform twenty-five feet of each in a walking fashion. Hold for three to five seconds with each step.

1. World's Greatest Stretch
2. Standing Superman Reach
3. Cross Body Knee Grab
4. Knee to Chest
5. Frankensteins
6. Alternating Toe Touches

Perform twenty-five repetitions of the following on each side.

7. Forward/Backward Leg Swings
8. Sideways Leg Swings

Core Stabilization and Strength (Chapter 8)

Perform two or three days a week. Pick two or three exercises from each category (Strength and Stabilization) for a total of four to six exercises per day. Select different exercises each day you perform your core strength and stabilization. Remember the tiered system of the exercises: beginner (B), intermediate (I), advanced (A), and expert (E). Work at the level that you are challenged at but able to control well. Progress this as you improve but do not forget about the more basic exercises. It is fun and creates good variety to revisit these every now and then.

For efficiency and overall benefit, try performing the exercises in a circuit. To do this, select two or three from each category and then pair them up. Complete the pair in an alternating fashion without taking a break. Rest for one to two minutes after a circuit and then begin the next circuit, again alternating between that pair.

Core Strength

<u>Clamshell Progression:</u> Two to four sets of fifteen to twenty-five repetitions
B—Clamshell
B—Reverse Clamshell
A—Super Clamshell
E—Super Duper Clamshell

<u>Resistance Band Walks:</u> Two to four sets of twenty-foot distance
B—Sideways Walk
I—Monster Walk
I—Train Tracks
A—Tandem Walk

<u>Leg Raises/Kicks:</u> Two to four sets of fifteen to twenty repetitions
B—Three Way Leg Raises
B—Donkey Kick
I—Steamboats
I—Sidelying Runner

<u>Squat Progression:</u> Two to three sets of ten to fifteen repetitions
B—Two Leg
I—Two Leg Suitcase
A—One Leg Step Down
E—One Leg Suitcase Squat

<u>RDL Progression:</u> Two to three sets of two to fifteen repetitions
B—Two Leg RDL with Stick
I—Two Leg Resisted RDL
A/E—Single Leg with or without Resistance
E—Airplane
*E—Nordic Curl

Core Stabilization

<u>Bridge Progression:</u> Two to four sets of ten to fifteen repetitions
B—Two Leg Bridge
I—Marching Bridge with Band
A—One Leg Bridge
E—One Leg Bridge with Physio Ball Hamstring Curl

<u>Plank Progression:</u> Three to five sets with a thirty to sixty second hold or a five to ten breath hold
B—Plank
I—Foot Walk Outs
A—Ball Plank
E—Stir the Pots
E—Ball Walk Out

<u>Side Plank Progression:</u> Three to five sets with a thirty- to sixty-second hold or a five to ten breath hold
B—Side Plank
I—Side Plank with Resisted Lowering
A—Side Plank Rotations

<u>Quadruped Progression:</u> Two to four sets of ten to fifteen repetitions or three to five repetitions holding for three to five breaths each
B—Leg Reach
I—Bird Dog
A—Bear Crawl

<u>Supine Progression:</u> Two to four sets of ten to fifteen repetitions or three to five repetitions holding for three to five breaths each
B—90/90 Holds
I—Leg Reach
A—Dying Bug
A—Ball Pinch Alternating Arm and Leg Reach

Half Kneel/Lunge Progression: The first position, the narrow half kneel hold, should be performed in two to four sets of thirty to sixty seconds a side, or perform five to ten breaths while holding a side. The other exercises are more repetition-based. For these, perform two to four sets of ten to fifteen repetitions per side.

B—Narrow Half Kneel Hold

I—Chops

A—Lunge Anti-Rotation Press

A—Knee Resisted Lunge

E—Lunge Ups

Standing Progression: Two to four sets of thirty to sixty second hold per side (or per direction for Helicopters)

B—Resisted Arm Swing

I—Resisted Knee Raises

I—Suitcase Carry

E—Helicopters

Running Mechanics Drills (Chapter 9)

Perform pre-running at least two days a week. Select three drills from the first grouping and vary this from day to day. Perform the second group in its entirety. The second group should be an extension of your warm-up, especially on harder training days.

Perform three repetitions of thirty to sixty seconds of the drills that are done in place (marked with *). Perform two to three laps of fifty feet or three to five laps of twenty-five feet of the other drills.

Group 1:
- Two Leg Segway*
- One Leg Segway*
- Core Controlled Arm Swing Progression*
- Wall Drill*

- Charging Bulls*
- Skater Hops
- 100 Ups*
- Band Running*
- Runner Hop
- Cadence Hopping*
- Running in Place*

Group 2:
- Butt Kicks
- High Knees
- Shuffle
- Karaoke
- Marching A
- Marching B
- Skipping A
- Skipping B
- Bounding
- Fall into Running and Striders

Acknowledgments

Thanks to:

Jodie, my wife, for supporting me through this endeavor and listening to me ramble about this for most of a year without much complaint. She's amazing!

Brayden and Mason, my energetic, fun-loving boys, who have shown me first-hand what natural-born runners look like and how core strength truly develops.

Scott Douglas, for encouraging me to take on this challenge and making my words sound better than they ever would have otherwise.

Erin Strout, for jumping in feet first to help clean up the chapters.

Steven Fairfield, for his patience and talent in taking such incredible photographs.

Rebecca Frey, for lending her skilled hand and artistic mind with the illustrations.

Steve Chabot and Shelby Kaplan, who were willing, fun, enthusiastic, and darn good-looking models.

Coach Ron Herman for teaching me mental toughness: how to walk the 2 x 4 and how to slay the dragon. Coach Marv Berkowitz for showing me the importance of running mechanics at an early age. Coach Jim Fisher for being there almost every day of my college years and helping to develop my independence.

My colleagues and patients, who help me to grow professionally every day and challenge my clinical reasoning.

And finally, my parents, who have taught me I can do anything I put my mind to.

About the Author

Daniel J. Frey, DPT, CMP, CSCS, is a well-known orthopedic and sports physical therapist based in Portland, Maine. Dan received his Doctor of Physical Therapy degree from the University of New England. Prior to this, he attended the University of Delaware, where he completed his Bachelor of Science degree in exercise physiology with minors in strength and conditioning and biology.

Dan specializes in the treatment of runners and has trained extensively in gait analysis and running biomechanics. He works regularly with a variety of patients, including recreational and professional athletes. While at UD, Dan competed at the Division I level in cross country, indoor track, and outdoor track, and was the captain of each team during his senior year. An avid runner, he has raced at distances ranging from 400 meters to 50 kilometers. He also enjoys spending time in the woods of Maine biking, climbing, skiing, and hiking.